The Kidneys and the Internal Environment

R. J. HARVEY,
Lecturer in Physiology
University of Bristol

CHAPMAN AND HALL
London
A HALSTED PRESS BOOK
JOHN WILEY & SONS
New York

First published 1974
by Chapman and Hall Ltd
11 New Fetter Lane, London EC4P 4EE

© 1974 R.J. Harvey

Typeset by E.W.C. Wilkins Ltd, London
and printed in Great Britain by
T. & A. Constable Ltd, Edinburgh

Library of Congress Cataloging in Publication Data

Harvey, Robert James.
    The kidneys and the internal environment.

    Bibliography: p.
    1. Kidneys. I. Title. [DNLM: 1. Body fluids—
Physiology. 2. Kidney—Physiology. WJ102 H342k 1974]
QP249.H37   612'.463   74—2776
ISBN 0—470—35775—4

Contents

Preface

This book owes its origin to my attempts to teach undergraduate students about the physiology of the kidneys and body fluids. I found that to increase my own knowledge and understanding of the subject it was necessary to begin from the basic chemical and physical principles which are involved in the physiology of the tissue fluids and the kidneys. The use of terms defined according to these basic principles provides a consistent nomenclature which is a considerable help in gaining a good understanding of the subject. This approach enables the student to avoid a great deal of the difficulty and confusion to which a descriptive approach and the use of the traditional misleading and inconsistent nomenclature inevitably lead [14].

I feel that an approach firmly based on an understanding of the basic physical and chemical processes and of the basic renal mechanisms offers a number of important advantages. These basic principles provide a reliable, logical and consistent framework around which further knowledge can be built, making the details much easier to learn and remember. When working outside the limits of one's certain knowledge, an extrapolation based on an understanding of the principles is much more likely to be right, or at least not seriously wrong, than one based on purely descriptive knowledge. A clear understanding of the principles which govern the way in which the body regulates the volume and composition of the internal environment is of considerable help to medical students and practitioners when they encounter patients with abnormal internal environments, and enables them to appreciate the likely origins and possible treatments for the abnormalities.

One disadvantage of the approach is that it does require the basic principles not only to be learnt, but to be thought about

until they are properly understood. Initially, this may require rather more effort than would be necessary merely to learn descriptive facts. However, once the basic principles have been mastered, a great deal of the material in the standard works on renal physiology and in original papers becomes much easier to evaluate and understand.

An attempt has been made to keep the book as short and simple as possible. Many statements are made without any, or with only very scanty, description of the evidence for them. Those topics which are treated in detail have been chosen because they were thought to provide good illustrations for particular aspects of the physiology, rather than because they are necessarily of special importance in themselves. For these reasons, this is not a comprehensive text book, but is intended to provide a solid framework upon which those who need more detailed knowledge can build.

I would like to thank my colleague, Dr. D.M. Armstrong, for his very helpful advice and criticism and for his encouragement throughout the writing of this book. I would also like to thank Miss C. Sharvelle for her help with the preparation of the manuscript.

Bristol,   R.J. Harvey
November 1973

1. Basic Principles

1.1 *Introduction*

In order to stay alive, all animals depend on many different chemical reactions taking place in their bodies. The overall rates and particularly the relative rates of these reactions must be very accurately controlled for the proper functioning of the animal as a whole. The rates of chemical reactions depend very critically upon the concentration of the reactants and on the temperature. The great majority of the various reactions in an animal take place within its cells, but the chemical composition and temperature of the inside of a cell is very much affected by the chemical composition and temperature of its environment. Claude Bernard recognized that, in higher animals, the environment of the cells is not at all the same as the environment outside the animal, but that it is what he called the *milieu intérieure*, which, in English, is called the *internal environment* [6]. For most cells, this is the extracellular fluid of the tissue within which the cell lies; so long as its state is maintained constant, what happens in the outside world need not affect what is going on in the cells.

This means that, whatever happens outside the animal, the cells are able to continue their operations under constant and optimum conditions. As Bernard said: 'the constancy of the internal environment is the requirement for a free and independent life'. All higher animals are able to control the chemical composition of their internal environment, that is of their extracellular fluid, very closely. This process is known as chemical homeostasis and the kidneys are very closely involved in it. Birds and mammals (and indeed some other animals) are able in addition to control the temperature of their internal environment, and

1

this gives them some advantage over lower animals, since it provides independence from the external environment in respect of another of the factors which alter the rates of reactions.

This book is about the physiology of the kidneys and the regulation of the internal environment in man and other mammals. The species on which the greatest amount of research has been done are man, dog and albino rat. Although work on many other species suggests that mammalian kidneys in general operate in basically the same way there are differences of detail between species, so that the contents of the book are likely not to apply to all mammals. Apart from anything else, different species cover a great range of sizes, so there are great quantitative differences of renal function between them. In order that quantitative measures of renal function should be consistent, they are quoted for man. However, not all men are the same size. It has been found in practice that, for normal young men, quantitative measures of renal function are most consistent from one subject to another when expressed in terms of the surface area of the body. Measures of renal function are commonly expressed in terms of a 'standard healthy young adult' who weighs 70 kg and has a surface area of 1.73 m^2. The measures quoted all apply to such a person unless otherwise stated.

In order that the composition of the internal environment shall remain constant, the quantities of the various substances which it contains must remain constant. All of these substances (or their metabolic precursors) occur in the diet, so that only if each substance leaves the internal environment at the same rate as it enters will the composition of the internal environment remain constant. For most animals, the composition of the diet, and hence the rate of input of the various substances, may change considerably from time to time and the homeostatic mechanisms which adjust the rates of output of the various substances via the kidneys have to maintain a very delicate dynamic balance between the rates of output and input of each substance. Because of this balance and because of the way in which some of the mechanisms may interact, it is only possible to understand what the kidneys do if they are studied in quantitative as well as in

qualitative terms. Such a study necessarily involves the use of numerical values and is made easier by the use of equations which show how the numerical values of various parameters are related to one another. Equations provide a very convenient and brief way of representing such relationships, but are often difficult to understand at first sight. For this reason an attempt has been made to reduce the number of equations used and to explain the significance of those which remain in words as well as symbols.

Another corollary of a quantitative treatment of the subject is the necessity to express measurements in units. There is no generally agreed system of units in use in physiology, although the use of SI units where appropriate is becoming almost universal. Unfortunately, there are a number of units which have been found to be very useful in physiology, but which do not directly correspond to any SI unit. To completely eliminate such units would be possible, but would probably create considerably more confusion than it would save. In this book, the recommendations of van Assendelft et $al.$ [2] have been followed and a number of 'non SI' units retained. The important ones are equivalents (see Section 1.2), the pH notation for hydrogen ion concentration (see Section 1.3) and mmHg for pressure (1 mmHg $\approx$ 133 N m^{-2}).

As an example of the sort of regulation of the internal environment which is necessary, consider the problems of someone such as a stoker, who does physical work in a hot environment. He will produce a considerable volume of sweat while he is working, the evaporation of which keeps his body temperature down, but also leads to the loss of water and salt (i.e. NaCl) from the body. This produces a fall in volume and a rise in osmotic pressure of the extracellular fluid. Drinking water will restore the volume but will tend to produce a fall in osmotic pressure. Eating some well-salted food will probably more than restore the salt content of the body, tending to produce an increase in osmotic pressure or an increase in volume of the extracellular fluid. The volume and composition of the internal environment remain remarkably constant under normal circumstances, despite all such factors which tend to change them.

Most of the mechanisms which control the constancy of the internal environment operate via the kidneys, so that a change in the internal environment leads to an alteration in the operation of the kidneys which tends to reverse the change. In order to appreciate the sort of regulation which the kidneys are capable of, it is necessary first to consider in detail what changes in the internal environment are likely to occur as a result of alterations in external circumstances. By next looking at the kidneys on their own, the effect alterations in their operation will have on the internal environment can be seen. Putting these two aspects together, it is possible to see the ways in which the kidneys are involved in keeping the internal environment constant despite changes in external conditions. In line with the above approach, the first chapter of this book deals with the basic principles underlying the chemical properties of the internal environment. The second chapter deals with the kidneys in isolation, while the two final chapters give an overall view of the way in which the volume and composition of the internal environment is maintained.

1.2 *Aqueous Solutions*

The extracellular fluid is a dilute solution of various chemical substances in water. Most of the chemical reactions described in this book take place in the body in dilute aqueous solution, so it will be as well to describe some of the relevant properties of such a solution. Many substances ionize completely in dilute solution: for example, sodium chloride splits up into sodium and chloride ions. This means that a solution made up of a mixture of ionized substances cannot be thought of as a mixture of the substances put in, but only of their constituent ions. For example, a mixture of sodium chloride and potassium nitrate solutions no longer contains these salts as such, but a mixture of sodium, potassium, chloride and nitrate ions. The different ions are effectively completely independent, the only proviso being that the total charge on the cations (or positively charged ions, in this example, Na^+ and K^+) must balance the total charge on the

anions (or negatively charged ions, i.e. Cl^- and NO_3^- here). The hair would literally stand on end as a result of the electrical potential produced by a difference in these totals much too small to measure with chemical techniques!

The concentration of a substance in aqueous solution is normally measured in terms of the number of molecules of the substance contained in unit quantity of the solution. The number of molecules is expressed in moles (i.e. gram-molecules) or millimoles, abbreviated to mol or mmol respectively. A solution is described as being n molar if it contains n moles of the solute in 1 kg of solution. Although concentrations should strictly speaking be expressed in terms of moles per kg of solution, they are in practice often measured in moles per litre. In the concentrations which are found in the tissue fluids etc. the difference is of no physiological significance and so will be ignored.

A universally used shorthand notation for the molar concentration of a substance is to enclose its chemical formula in square brackets. For example, [NaCl] represents a concentration of sodium chloride in moles per litre (or kg) of solution. For substances which ionize in solution, especially when a number of different ions are present, it is usual to deal with the concentration of each ion separately, e.g. $[Na^+]$ and $[Cl^-]$. These concentrations may be expressed in moles, but for some purposes it is more useful to consider the concentration of charge associated with a particular ion rather than the concentration of particles of the ion. The concentration of ionic charge is expressed in equivalents per litre, which can be thought of as the concentration of charge measured in terms of the charge on an electron, and expressed in moles per litre. Milliequivalents are conventionally abbreviated to mEq, and, here, Eq will be used for equivalents. The usefulness of equivalents arises from the fact that in any solution the total number of anionic (negative) charges must exactly balance the total number of cationic (positive) charges in order to preserve electrical neutrality. For univalent ions, moles and equivalents are the same, but for divalent ions (e.g. Ca^{++}, SO_4^{--}), each mole represents two equivalents (and so on for ions of higher valency). 1 mole of sodium sulphate (Na_2SO_4)

in solution gives 2 moles of sodium ions, but only 1 mole of sulphate ions. However, the number of equivalents of anions and cations balance, since there are 2 equivalents of each. For some ions, the number of equivalents is not an exact multiple of the number of moles and may vary depending on other factors in the solution. (For instance, 1 mole of phosphate ions represents 1.8 equivalents when the pH of the solution is 7.4, but only 1.01 equivalent if the pH is reduced to 4.8 — see Sections 1.5 and 4.8).

The above units measure the concentrations of substances, and the rate at which a substance in unit volume of solution takes part in a chemical reaction depends on its concentration. Equations for the rates of reactions are usually expressed in terms of the concentrations of the reacting substances, e.g. equation (1.2). In this case what really matters is not the amount of the substance in the solution but the amount available for reaction, which is termed its activity and which may be less than its concentration. Although under certain circumstances the activity of an ion may be very much less than its concentration in a solution (particularly in a concentrated solution), for the ions whose reactions are going to be discussed, the activity and the concentration are so nearly the same that concentrations can be used without introducing any significant error. (This does not apply to all ions in the plasma. For example, the activity of calcium ions is normally very much less than the calcium concentration, because much of the calcium present is in combination rather than as ions).

1.3 *Dissociation of Water*

Water is, in a sense, an unstable substance. Water molecules spontaneously split up into hydrogen ions and hydroxyl ions. This is represented by the equation:

$$H_2O \longrightarrow H^+ + OH^-$$

Both the hydrogen ions and the hydroxyl ions so formed become hydrated by associating with undissociated water molecules, to form a rather loose complex. No proper chemical bond is formed,

and each actual ion can readily transfer from one water molecule (or group of water molecules) to another. The hydration of the ions does not have any great effect on their chemical affinities, except that they are to some extent 'protected' from other reactants by their associated water molecules so that it is likely to reduce the rate of their reactions somewhat. In the following account, the water molecules associated with the ions will not be specifically mentioned again, but when 'hydrogen ions' or 'hydroxyl ions' are referred to, this refers to the hydrated ions (together with the exceedingly small number of ions which exist in the unhydrated form).

At a constant temperature, any particular water molecule has a constant probability of dissociating within a given time interval, so that the rate at which hydrogen and hydroxyl ions are formed increases directly with the total number of water molecules. The rate of dissociation in a unit volume of solution will be proportional to the water concentration. This relationship may be expressed as an equation:

$$\text{Rate of dissociation} = K[\text{H}_2\text{O}] \qquad (1.1)$$

(where K is a constant. The actual probability of dissociation changes with temperature, so the rate of dissociation per unit volume and hence the value of K will also change with temperature). If this dissociation continued indefinitely, it would be expected that eventually all the water molecules would become dissociated. However, when a hydrogen ion and a hydroxyl ion collide in a suitable way in the course of their random thermal movements, they will recombine to form a water molecule:

$$\text{H}^+ + \text{OH}^- \longrightarrow \text{H}_2\text{O}$$

The rate at which this occurs will obviously depend on the total number of collisions between the two types of ion, since collisions which lead on to combination will be a certain proportion of the total collisions. For any given hydrogen ion, the chance of its colliding with a hydroxyl ion will depend on the concentration of hydroxyl ions. The total number of hydrogen ion–hydroxyl ion collisions per unit volume will therefore depend on the

concentration of hydroxyl ions multiplied by the number of hydrogen ions per unit volume, or, in other words, on the product of their concentrations. This can also be expressed in an equation:

$$\text{Rate of formation of water} = k\,[\text{OH}^-]\,[\text{H}^+] \qquad (1.2)$$

(where k is another constant).

If one could start with pure and completely undissociated water, it would immediately start to dissociate at the rate given by equation (1.1). However, as soon as hydrogen ions and hydroxyl ions are formed, they will start to recombine at the rate given by equation (1.2). At first the recombination will be very slow, as the concentrations of the ions will be very low, but as the concentrations build up, the rate of recombination will increase. Eventually, a state of equilibrium will be reached when the rate of recombination becomes equal to the rate of dissociation. After this, no further changes in the concentrations will occur, even though dissociation and recombination are still continuously taking place. At equilibrium, the rates of the two reactions are equal, so:

$$\text{rate of dissociation} = \text{rate of formation}$$

and so, from equations (1.1) and (1.2):

$$K[\text{H}_2\text{O}] = k\,[\text{H}^+]\,[\text{OH}^-]$$

or

$$\frac{[\text{H}^+]\,[\text{OH}^-]}{[\text{H}_2\text{O}]} = K/k$$

This is the usual way of expressing the equilibrium concentrations of the substances taking part in a reversible reaction, as given by the Law of Mass Action. However, in the case of water it is more convenient to express the equilibrium as:

$$[\text{H}^+]\,[\text{OH}^-] = K/k\,[\text{H}_2\text{O}]$$

In this case, the concentrations of hydrogen ions and hydroxyl ions are always very much less than the concentration of water, so that the concentration of water effectively does not change. (It is 55.5 mol l^{-1} in pure water.) The three quantities on the right of this equation are then all constants and can be combined

to form another constant – here written as K'. Thus:

$$[H^+][OH^-] = K' \qquad (1.3)$$

K' is called the dissociation constant of water and has a value of 10^{-14} at 25 °C. For pure water, the number of hydrogen ions and hydroxyl ions must be the same, so that:

$$\text{as} \quad [H^+][OH^-] = 10^{-14},$$

$$[H^+][H^+] = 10^{-14}$$

from which both $[H^+]$ and $[OH^-]$ are 10^{-7} (mol l^{-1}).

Addition to pure water of various substances known as acids or bases (see Section 1.5) may alter the hydrogen ion and hydroxyl ion concentrations, but the product of their concentrations remains the same, so that if the concentration of one rises, that of the other must fall. Such acids or bases must be ionized substances as the total number of anions and cations in the solution must balance, and the numbers of hydrogen ions and hydroxyl ions no longer do so. The effect on the hydrogen and hydroxyl ion concentrations of adding acids and bases is conventionally expressed in terms of the final concentration of hydrogen ions in the solution. Two different types of notation are used to express this concentration, either moles/litre (mol l^{-1}), in the usual way for other substances, or in pH units.

1.4 *What is pH?*

The pH notation is simply a way of expressing the concentration of hydrogen ions in a solution, but which uses a different notation from the more usual way of expressing concentrations in moles or equivalents per litre. It was originally introduced to avoid the use of many zeros or large (negative) powers of 10 which would be necessary if moles/litre were expressed directly. pH is defined as 'the negative logarithm to base 10 of the hydrogen ion concentration of a solution in moles/litre'. In other words if the hydrogen ion concentration of a solution is 2 mEq l^{-1}, this is a concentration of 2×10^{-3} Eq l^{-1} or $1/(5 \times 10^2)$ Eq l^{-1}. The logarithm of 5×10^2

is (very nearly) 2.7, so the logarithm of $1/(5 \times 10^2)$ is -2.7, so that the pH of the solution is 2.7. It is useful to remember that a change of pH of 1 unit represents a tenfold change of hydrogen ion concentration and that a change of 0.3 of a unit represents (very nearly) a twofold change. It has been suggested [10] that it would be simpler not to use the pH notation at all, but to express the concentrations directly in mol (or Eq) l^{-1}, and it is, indeed, somewhat easier to visualize the latter notation. However the pH notation does have a number of advantages, some of which are set out below.

Since the pH scale is logarithmic, a certain change of the value of the pH of a solution represents a change of the actual hydrogen ion concentration by a certain ratio rather than by a certain absolute quantity. When the properties of buffer systems are considered (Section 1.5), it will be seen that a certain proportional change (e.g. a doubling) in the hydrogen ion concentration is associated with the same change in the ratio of the concentrations of the two components of the buffer system. It is rather easier to calculate the changes in the concentrations of the buffer components (and of hydrogen ions) if the pH notation is used for the hydrogen ion concentration.

From the Law of Mass Action, the magnitude of the chemical effects of changes of hydrogen ion concentration is related to the proportional change in the concentration and therefore to the numerical change in pH rather than to the absolute change in terms of Eq litre^{-1}. Moreover the biological effects of changes in the hydrogen ion concentration of the extracellular fluid also appear to depend on the change as measured in pH units rather than in absolute terms. Thus the normal human arterial plasma pH is about 7.4 (40×10^{-9} Eq l^{-1}) and the limits compatible with life are from pH 7.0 to 7.8, i.e. $\pm$ 0.4 pH units, which represents a range from 100 to 16×10^{-9} Eq l^{-1}, or an increase of 60 but a decrease of only 24×10^{-9} Eq l^{-1}. Although this is a difference in absolute terms of only 84×10^{-9} Eq l^{-1}, it is an eightfold change in concentration, which is many times greater than the proportional changes in, for example, the sodium or potassium concentrations of the extracellular fluid which are

compatible with life.

Although the plasma hydrogen ion concentration varies only over quite narrow limits, the hydrogen ion concentrations of various other physiological fluids in mammals range from about 0.1 Eq l^{-1} to 0.000 000 003 Eq l^{-1} (or 10^{-1} to 3×10^{-9} Eq l^{-1}), but using the pH notation, this range extends only from 1 to 8.5.

pH (or rather the activity of hydrogen ions) is normally measured by using a pH meter. A pH meter depends on the properties of a hollow electrode made of special glass which is permeable to hydrogen ions, but not to other ions. The meter measures the equilibrium potential across the glass membrane between the unknown solution outside the electrode and a solution of known hydrogen ion concentration inside the electrode. The potential depends on the ratio of the hydrogen ion concentrations (see Section 1.8), so whatever the pH, a given change in pH produces (or in theory should produce) a given change in the voltage measured by the pH meter, while a given change of hydrogen ion concentration does not. It is very much easier to calibrate the meter in terms of pH rather than in terms of concentration.

Thus, under some circumstances, hydrogen ion concentration is most conveniently expressed in the pH notation, while under others the concentration in Eq l^{-1} is more suitable; there are many advantages in retaining both notations, and they will both be used hereafter.

1.5 *Acids, Bases and Buffers*

Water spontaneously ionizes as described in Section 1.3. The dissociation constant for water at 25 °C is 10^{-14}, so that for pure water:

$$[H^+] = [OH^-] = \sqrt{10^{-14}} = 10^{-7}$$

Now the logarithm (to base 10) of 10^{-7} is -7, so that the pH of pure water at 25 °C is 7.

If a small amount of an acid (as defined below) is added to pure water, then the concentration of hydrogen ions will rise.

Some of the hydrogen ions added will combine with hydroxyl ions, so that the hydroxyl ion concentration will fall (the product of the hydrogen and hydroxyl ion concentrations must remain constant). Similarly, addition of a base (or alkali) to pure water will cause the hydroxyl ion concentration to rise and the hydrogen ion concentration to fall.

A solution which contains more hydrogen ions than hydroxyl ions is said to be acid and one which contains more hydroxyl ions than hydrogen ions is said to be alkaline, and one which contains the same number of each is said to be neutral. Thus at 25 °C a neutral solution has a pH of 7. However, the dissociation of water varies with temperature, and at 37 °C:

$$[H^+][OH^-] = 10^{-13.6}$$

so if $$[H^+] = [OH^-],$$

then $$[H^+][H^+] = 10^{-13.6},$$

from which $$[H^+] = \sqrt{10^{-13.6}} = 10^{-6.8}$$

so that a neutral solution has a hydrogen ion concentration of $10^{-6.8}$ Eq litre^{-1} or a pH of 6.8.

The terms acid and base have precise chemical definitions. However, for physiological purposes it is convenient to paraphrase and slightly simplify these definitions and to define an acid as a substance which in solution tends to make a neutral solution acid, either by releasing hydrogen ions into the solution or by removing hydroxyl ions. Conversely, a base is a substance which tends to make the solution alkaline, either by releasing hydroxyl ions or by removing hydrogen ions. Many substances are neutral (i.e. neither acids nor bases) either because they do not produce any significant number of either hydrogen or hydroxyl ions in solution (e.g. glucose) or because they produce equal numbers of both (e.g. water). Acids and bases are described as being of various strengths (from 'very strong' to 'very weak') depending essentially on the number of hydrogen ions which they release into (or remove from) solution for each potentially available hydrogen ion (or hydroxyl ion) added to the solution. For instance hydro-chloric acid is a very strong acid because in dilute solution the

reaction $HCl \rightleftharpoons H^+ + Cl^-$ proceeds almost completely to the right, so that virtually all the potentially available hydrogen ions are released into the solution. Similarly sodium hydroxide is a very strong base because the reaction $NaOH \rightleftharpoons Na^+ + OH^-$ also proceeds almost completely to the right. On the other hand, sodium chloride is effectively neutral because it dissociates virtually completely in a dilute solution into equal numbers of sodium ions and chloride ions, which are extremely weak acids and bases respectively. Sodium ions act as a very weak acid because they have a very small but nevertheless finite tendency to combine with hydroxyl ions and remove them from solution, and chloride ions similarly have a very small tendency to combine with hydrogen ions. However these two ions are so weak that for all practical purposes they can be considered neutral. Between these two extremes are a whole range of acids and bases of different strengths.

When a strong acid is added to a solution, all the hydrogen ions which the acid contains are released, but not all of them necessarily remain free (although this is almost true when the acid is added to pure water). For example, if 10^{-4} mol of strong acid (e.g. hydrochloric) are added to pure water to make up a litre of solution, the hydrogen ion concentration of the mixture will (at 25 °C) be governed by equation (1.3), i.e.:

$$[H^+] [OH^-] = 10^{-14}$$

so that as the hydrogen ion concentration rises, the hydroxyl ion concentration must fall. For each hydroxyl ion that disappears, a hydrogen ion also disappears since

$$OH^- + H^+ \rightleftharpoons H_2O$$

The final hydrogen ion concentration may be calculated by considering the two things which may happen to the added hydrogen ions — either they may remain free in solution or they may combine with hydroxyl ions. Let these quantities be y and z Eq respectively. The final hydrogen ion concentration will then be $(10^{-7} + y)$ and the hydroxyl ion concentration will be $(10^{-7} - z)$.

From equation (1.3):

$$(10^{-7} + y)(10^{-7} - z) = 10^{-14}$$

and $y + z = 10^{-4}$ (the number of hydrogen ions added).

This gives 2 simultaneous equations which can be solved for y and z, which allows the final hydrogen ion concentration to be calculated. It is almost exactly 10^{-4}, so that the final pH is 4.000 (to 4 significant figures).

If a weak acid is added to water, the change in pH is smaller than when an equivalent amount of strong acid is added, because some of the potentially available hydrogen ions are not released into the solution. For example, acetic acid (here written HAc, for simplicity) in solution dissociates as follows:

$$HAc \rightleftharpoons H^+ + Ac^-$$

but the reaction does not go to completion, so an equilibrium is reached such that:

$$\frac{[H^+]\,[Ac^-]}{[HAc]} = K \qquad (1.4)$$

where K in this case is about 2×10^{-5} (or $10^{-4.7}$) at 25 °C.

If 10^{-4} mol of acetic acid are added to a litre of pure water, the the final hydrogen ion concentration is about 3.58×10^{-5} Eq l^{-1} (corresponding to a pH of 4.45) or less than half the concentration produced by an equivalent amount of strong acid. The balance of the hydrogen ions are still combined with acetate ions as undissociated acetic acid. The fact that acetic acid dissociates relatively little implies that acetate ions combine readily with hydrogen ions, so that acetate ions act as a base, and as a result a solution of sodium acetate has a pH greater than 7.

If acetic acid and acetate ions are present in a solution, there are some potentially available hydrogen ions in the acetic acid and also some acetate ions which readily combine with hydrogen ions. If hydrogen ions as strong acid are added, some of the acetate ions will each take up a hydrogen ion reducing the change of actual hydrogen ion concentration. Similarly, if strong alkali is added, some of the hydroxyl ions will combine with some of

the potentially available hydrogen ions in previously undissociated molecules of acetic acid. The presence of the acetate ions and acetic acid thus reduces the change of pH that would have occurred with the addition of strong acid or alkali, and they are said to 'buffer' the solution. A buffer may be defined as a substance which in solution acts in such a way that if strong acid (or alkali) is added, the change of pH is less than it would have been had the buffer not been there. Substances which act as buffers are weak acids or bases and their associated ions.

To take an example of buffering, consider what happens when strong acid is added to an acetate solution with an initial pH of 7. If the initial acetate ion concentration is 10^{-1} mol l^{-1} (of dissociated ions), the concentration of undissociated acetic acid can be calculated.

$$\frac{[H^+] [Ac^-]}{[HAc]} = 10^{-4.7} \text{ from equation (1.4)}$$

$[H^+]$ has been set to 10^{-7}, and $[Ac^-]$ to 10^{-1}, so that substituting these values into the equation, $[HAc] = 10^{-3.3}$. When 10^{-4} Eq of hydrogen ions (as strong acid) is now added, some will combine with the acetate ions to produce acetic acid (x Eq, which will remove x Eq of acetate ions from solution to create x Eq of acetic acid), some will remain as free hydrogen ions, (y Eq) and a few will combine with hydroxyl ions to form water (z Eq, which will remove z Eq of hydroxyl ions from solution). Now, from the equilibrium for water — equation (1.3),

$$[10^{-7} + y] [10^{-7} - z] = 10^{-14}$$

and, from the equilibrium for acetic acid — equation (1.4),

$$\frac{[10^{-7} + y] [10^{-1} - x]}{[10^{-3.3} + x]} = 10^{-4.7}$$

and

$$x + y + z = 10^{-4} - \text{the number of hydrogen ions added.}$$

These form a set of 3 simultaneous equations from which x, y and z can be calculated. The hydrogen ion concentration is approx 1.2×10^{-7} corresponding to a pH of about 6.92. Thus,

in this particular example, the presence of the acetate ions has reduced the pH change from 3 units to 0.08 units or reduced the change in hydrogen ion concentration by a factor of about 800.

A method similar to the one used for the particular example above can be used to calculate the changes that occur for any buffer when acid or alkali is added to the solution, whatever the hydrogen ion concentration. However, the calculation is rather tedious, and if the change in pH is relatively small, a good approximation to the final pH can be obtained by a much simpler method, as described below. Acetic acid will again be used as an example. Equation (1.4) gives:

$$\frac{[H^+]\,[Ac^-]}{[HAc]} = K$$

Dividing both sides by $[Ac^-]$ and multiplying by $[HAc]$, this becomes:

$$[H^+] = K\,\frac{[HAc]}{[Ac^-]} \tag{1.5}$$

Taking logarithms (to base 10) of both sides,

$$\log [H^+] = \log K + \log [HAc] - \log [Ac^-]$$

Changing the signs

$$-\log [H^+] = -\log K - \log [HAc] + \log [Ac^-]$$

or

$$pH = -\log K + \log [Ac^-] - \log [HAc].$$

Since the difference of two logarithms gives the logarithm of the quotient,

$$\log [Ac^-] - \log [HAc] \text{ is the same as } \log \frac{[Ac^-]}{[HAc]}$$

Using a notation analagous to the use of pH as a symbol for $-\log [H^+]$, pK is commonly used as a symbol for $-\log K$, so that:

$$pH = pK + \log \frac{[Ac^-]}{[HAc]} \tag{1.6}$$

This is a very useful relationship which is known as the Henderson–Hasselbalch equation and which applies, with

appropriate values of pK and concentrations of the relevant substances, to any acid or base and its associated ions in aqueous solution.

Substituting the values in the above example into equation (1.6)

$$7 = 4.7 + \log \frac{[10^{-1}]}{[10^{-3.3}]}$$

The change of pH produced by adding acid can now be calculated by assuming that all the added hydrogen ions combine with the buffer. Thus, for the above example, after adding the acid,

$$pH = 4.7 + \log \frac{[10^{-1} - 10^{-4}]}{[10^{-3.3} + 10^{-4}]}$$

from which (to 3 significant figures)

$$pH = 6.92$$

This is the same result (to 3 significant figures) as is given by the more accurate method described earlier. That the approximation is good depends on the fact that the number of the added hydrogen ions remaining free is a very small proportion of their total number, the great majority combining with the buffer. However, this is no longer true when the change in hydrogen ion concentration is large, when a significant fraction of the added hydrogen ions remains uncombined or combines with hydroxyl ions rather than with the buffer. Since the pH of the internal environment fluctuates only within narrow limits, the approximation is nearly always good enough for use in physiological calculations.

Equations (1.5) and (1.6) show that for any buffer system, the ratio between the 'buffer base' and 'buffer acid' concentrations (acetate ions and unionized acetic acid respectively in this particular example) is set by the hydrogen ion concentration (and vice versa), so that, if either one is altered, the other must change appropriately. In a solution containing more than one buffer system, there can only be one value of hydrogen ion concentration and this determines the individual ratios of the concentrations for each system of buffer base and buffer acid, the

individual values of the ratios depending on the individual pKs (i.e. dissociation constants) for each system. Since each buffer system operates independently apart from this, the total number of hydrogen ions buffered for a given change in pH is the sum of the hydrogen ions taken up by each individual buffer system. Thus, the total 'buffering capacity' is the sum of that provided by each individual buffer system in the solution.

The effectiveness of a particular buffer system depends both on its concentration and on the ratio of the acid and the basic components initially present (and hence on the initial pH.). Obviously the greater the concentration of a buffer, the more hydrogen ions it will remove from solution for a given change in the (free) hydrogen ion concentration, so that addition of a certain quantity of acid will produce a smaller change of pH. In fact, doubling the concentration of the buffer will approximately halve the pH change for the addition of a given amount of acid (or alkali).

The effect of the initial pH (or the ratio of buffer base to buffer acid) on the buffering is a little harder to visualize, but it is easy to see that once all (or nearly all) the base form has been converted to the acid form, no more hydrogen ions can be taken up so no more buffering can occur. The situation can be analysed rather more rigorously. From the Henderson–Hasselbalch equation (e.g. for acetate again):

$$pH = pK + \log \frac{[Ac^-]}{[HAc]} = pK + \log [Ac^-] - \log [HAc]$$

In the course of buffering, for each hydrogen ion removed from solution, one acetate ion disappears and one molecule of acetic acid appears. If the solution is initially made up with C moles per litre of sodium acetate (and no acetic acid) then $[Ac^-] + [HAc] = C$. Therefore if x moles litre^{-1} of hydrogen ions have been buffered, (rather than added) the concentration of acetic acid is x and of acetate ions is $(C - x)$, so:

$$pH = pK + \log (C - x) - \log (x)$$

This equation gives the relationship between the pH and the amount of acid buffered (x). The rate of change of pH with x

can be obtained by differentiating with respect to x:

$$\frac{\mathrm{dpH}}{\mathrm{d}x} = -\frac{1}{(C-x)} - \frac{1}{x}$$

This is negative for all possible values of x (i.e. between 0 and C), which is not unexpected, since the pH does fall with the addition of acid. It is also never zero, which illustrates the fact that addition of acid always does produce some change in pH, however much buffer is present.

The actual magnitude of the rate of change of pH with x will be given by:

$$\mathrm{Rate} = \frac{1}{(C-x)} + \frac{1}{x}$$

This will be very large either when x is very small (when the buffer is nearly all as acetate ions) so that $1/x$ becomes very large, or when x is very nearly equal to C (when it is nearly all acetic acid) so that $1/(C-x)$ becomes very large. At these points, the buffering will be very ineffective. The buffering will be most effective when the rate of change is least, which is in fact when $x = C/2$. Buffering is thus most effective when half of the buffer is in its basic form and half in its acidic form.

At this point,

$$\mathrm{pH} = \mathrm{p}K + \log\frac{C/2}{C/2} = \mathrm{p}K + \log 1 = \mathrm{p}K.$$

This means that acetate is most effective as a buffer at a pH of 4.7.

To take some specific examples, imagine a solution containing 1 mole of acetate (counting both acetic acid and acetate ions) per litre. If 1 mEq per litre of hydrogen ions as strong acid is added at various initial pH s, the changes in pH produced are as follows:

Initial pH	$\dfrac{[\mathrm{Ac}^-]}{[\mathrm{HAc}]}$	Final pH	Change in pH	Change in pH without any buffer
2.700	1/100	2.663	0.037	0.177
3.700	1/10	3.695	0.005	0.779
4.700	1	4.698	0.002	1.709
5.700	10	5.695	0.005	2.701
6.700	100	6.656	0.044	3.700

This again shows that buffering is most effective when the pH is equal to the pK of the buffer system, and it also shows that its effectiveness begins to fall off rather rapidly when the ratio of buffer base to acid is outside the range $1:10 - 10:1$.

1.6 *Proteins and their Buffering Properties*

Proteins are large molecules made up of amino-acids linked together to form peptide chains. Many amino-acids have groups at their 'non-peptide' end (i.e. the end away from the chain of peptide bonds in the protein molecule) which in solution can give off or take up hydrogen ions so that proteins may act as both acids and bases simultaneously: each of these groups has its own particular dissociation constant. (In the following equations, R represents the non-peptide end of a particular amino-acid and Prot represents the remainder of the protein molecule.)

$$HR\text{-Prot} \rightleftharpoons H^+ + R^-\text{-Prot}$$

or for other types of group:

$$HR^+\text{-Prot} \rightleftharpoons H^+ + R\text{-Prot}$$

The equilibrium for the reaction involving first type of group is:

$$\frac{[H^+]\,[R^-\text{-Prot}]}{[HR\text{-Prot}]} = k$$

This relationship can also be expressed in the format of the Henderson—Hasselbalch equation (equation 1.6):

$$pH = pk + \log \frac{[R^-\text{-Prot}]}{[HR\text{-Prot}]}$$

However the relationship is expressed, the important thing is that the tendency for a hydrogen ion to be combined with these groups will increase as the hydrogen ion concentration rises, i.e. as the pH falls. Since the hydrogen ions are positively charged, those groups which have combined with a hydrogen ion will lose their negative charge (or gain a positive charge). This means that the distribution of charges on the protein molecule will change

with pH and this will affect the electrostatic forces between the various groups which will in turn alter their positions relative to one another and so change the precise 3-dimensional form of the molecule. Since the activity of many enzymes seems to depend very critically on the relative positions of various parts of the molecule, the activity of an enzyme is likely to be affected by pH. An obvious example of this is provided by digestive enzymes. Pepsin is an effective proteolytic enzyme only at pH levels below about 4 while trypsin is most effective at a pH of about 8.

Another type of effect on the properties of a protein molecule which alteration of its charge distribution may have is demonstrated by haemoglobin. Here, the molecular shape and its chemical properties are altered when the haem groups take up oxygen. This alters the dissociation constants of the acidic and basic groups on the rest of the molecule in such a way that oxyhaemoglobin is a 'stronger' acid (i.e. a greater proportion of its ionizable hydrogen atoms are in solution as hydrogen ions at a given pH) than reduced haemoglobin. This works both ways, since when some of the acidic or basic groups take up hydrogen ions, this alters the charge distribution on the molecule so that the affinity of the haem groups for oxygen is reduced, so that some oxygen will be released. This is the basis for the so-called Bohr shift, which is the change in the haemoglobin-oxygen dissociation curve with change in pH. This property of haemoglobin means that the presence of an increased concentration of carbonic acid derived from the carbon dioxide produced by respiring cells leads to increased dissociation of oxygen from the haemoglobin so making the oxygen available where it is being used. The reduced haemoglobin then combines with many of the hydrogen ions derived from the carbonic acid, so minimizing the difference in pH between arterial and venous plasma. (For further details see Chapter 1 of ref. 13).

Most of the proteins in the plasma (and in cells) have a greater number of groups which give off hydrogen ions into solution as the pH rises, leaving negatively charged 'basic' groups behind, than they have of groups which take up hydrogen ions to become positively charged as the pH falls. Thus at the normal pH of the

plasma (and the intracellular fluid), the molecules are negatively charged. The different groups will usually all have different dissociation constants, but on most protein molecules, there are many groups with pK values fairly close to the normal value of pH of the body fluids. This means that a small change (e.g. a fall) in pH will lead to many of the groups taking up hydrogen ions from solution. Because of this, many more hydrogen ions will have been added to the solution than remain as free hydrogen ions. The proteins are thus making the change of (free) hydrogen ion concentration less than it would have been if they were not there and they are therefore acting as buffers.

Proteins are extremely important buffers in the plasma and within cells. In the plasma, the greater part of any added hydrogen ions are taken up by the plasma proteins and the haemoglobin in the red blood cells and only a small part by the non-protein buffers (i.e. phosphate and bicarbonate ions). However, although bicarbonate ions play a relatively small part in the chemical buffering of the plasma they are extremely important in the 'physiological buffering' which, except in the very short term, is a more powerful mechanism for minimizing changes in plasma pH, as described in the next Section.

1.7 *The Bicarbonate Buffer System*

The bicarbonate buffer system is extremely important in the body, but is a little more complicated than the acetate buffer system which has been used to illustrate the general properties of buffer systems. The reactions concerned depend on the properties of carbonic acid, which may split up into a hydrogen ion and a bicarbonate ion, or into carbon dioxide and water.

and:
$$HCO_3^- + H^+ \rightleftharpoons H_2CO_3 \qquad (1.7)$$
$$H_2CO_3 \rightleftharpoons H_2O + CO_2 \qquad (1.8)$$

In the absence of catalysts, the latter reaction takes place slowly and requires several minutes to come to equilibrium. This does not, of course, affect the position of equilibrium, but only the

speed with which it is reached following a change in the concentration of one of the components. For the equilibrium of the reaction represented by equation (1.7):

$$\frac{[H^+]\,[HCO_3^-]}{[H_2CO_3]} = k \tag{1.9}$$

and, in the format of the Henderson–Hasselbalch equation (equation 1.6)

$$pH = pk + \log\frac{[HCO_3^-]}{[H_2CO_3]} \tag{1.10}$$

For the reaction of equation (1.8)

$$\frac{[H_2CO_3]}{[H_2O]\,[CO_2]} = k'$$

Rearranging (by multiplying both sides by $[H_2O]$ and $[CO_2]$)

$$[H_2CO_3] = k'[H_2O]\,[CO_2]$$

Since in dilute solution $[H_2O]$ is as near constant as makes no difference, it can be incorporated into the equilibrium constant, so that:

$$[H_2CO_3] = k''[CO_2] \tag{1.11}$$

From Henry's law relating to the solubility of gases in fluids, the quantity of CO_2 in solution is directly proportional to the partial pressure of CO_2 in the gas with which the solution is in equilibrium. Thus:

$$[CO_2] = \alpha P_{CO_2} \tag{1.12}$$

(where P_{CO_2} is the partial pressure of CO_2, usually measured in mmHg, and α is the solubility constant of CO_2, measured in mol l^{-1} mmHg^{-1}; this changes with temperature, like most of the other constants considered). Thus, combining (1.11) and (1.12):

$$[H_2CO_3] = k''\alpha P_{CO_2}$$

Inserting this value for $[H_2CO_3]$ into equation (1.10):

$$pH = pk + \log\frac{[HCO_3^-]}{k''\alpha P_{CO_2}}$$

k'' can be separated from the right hand expression:

$$pH = pk - \log k'' + \log \frac{[HCO_3^-]}{\alpha P_{CO_2}}$$

pk and $(-\log k'')$ are both constant, so they can be combined to make another constant, here called pK.
Thus:

$$pH = pK + \log \frac{[HCO_3^-]}{\alpha P_{CO_2}} \qquad (1.13)$$

The value of pK in equation (1.13) is about 6.1 at 37 °C. This means that at the normal (human) plasma and extracellular fluid pH of 7.4, the value of $\log [HCO_3^-]/\alpha P_{CO_2}$ must be 1.3, so that the actual ratio is 20 (antilog of 1.3). In round figures, (chosen to simplify the arithmetic) the actual concentrations usually observed in the arterial plasma in man are 24 mmol l^{-1} for $[HCO_3^-]$ and 1.2 mmol l^{-1} for $[CO_2]$. Since α is approx. 0.00003 mol l^{-1} mmHg^{-1} (or 0.03 mmol l^{-1} mmHg^{-1}), this corresponds to a P_{CO_2} of 40 mmHg. As blood passes through the lungs, the plasma comes into equilibrium with the gas in the alveoli, so that the partial pressure of CO_2 here must also be 40 mmHg.

The P_{CO_2} in the alveolar gas depends on the rate of production of CO_2 and on the rate at which the gas in the alveoli is being replaced by fresh gas from the outside air. This rate will be referred to as the alveolar ventilation and depends on the total respiratory exchange, after allowing for the gas which is merely ventilating the 'dead space' of the respiratory system. When the body is in a steady state, carbon dioxide will be leaving the alveoli in the expired air at the same rate at which it is being produced by metabolism. The quantity leaving the body in unit time $(Q\ l\ min^{-1})$ must therefore be the same as the quantity produced in unit time, and is contained in the volume making up the alveolar ventilation $(V\ l\ min^{-1})$ in unit time. Thus the proportion of carbon dioxide in the alveolar gas must be Q/V. The partial pressure of carbon dioxide to which this corresponds will be given by:

$$P_{CO_2} = Q/V\ 760\ \text{mmHg (at sea level)}$$

If the rate of production of CO_2 (Q) remains constant, then the P_{CO_2} at equilibrium must be inversely proportional to the alveolar ventilation.

Since the ratio of bicarbonate to carbon dioxide in the plasma is a long way from 1 it would be expected to make it a not very efficient buffer system (as described above). However, because of 'physiological buffering' it is much better than would be expected on this basis. Physiological buffering depends on the P_{CO_2} being rapidly adjusted by the respiratory system and $[HCO_3^-]$ more slowly adjusted by the kidneys. These two mechanisms can therefore adjust the ratio of bicarbonate to carbon dioxide and alter the pH of the plasma and hence of the extracellular fluid as a whole.

If 1 mmol l^{-1} of strong acid is added to a bicarbonate solution made up with the same pH and bicarbonate concentration as the plasma, then, to a first approximation:

$$pH = 6.1 + \log\frac{(24 - 1)}{(1.2 + 1)} \qquad (1.14)$$

$$= 6.1 + \log\frac{23}{2.2}$$

$$= 6.1 + \log 10.05$$

$$= 7.12$$

The $[CO_2]$ has now gone up to 2.2 mmol l^{-1}, and the P_{CO_2} in equilibrium with this is about 73 mmHg. This rise in P_{CO_2} is due to the CO_2 produced from the bicarbonate ions which have combined with hydrogen ions, and, even with no change in the alveolar ventilation, it would cause an increase in the rate at which CO_2 leaves the body. The rate of excretion would now exceed the rate of metabolic CO_2 production, so the P_{CO_2} would rapidly drop back to 40 mmHg (and the $[CO_2]$ to 1.2 mmol l^{-1}) when equilibrium would again be reached.

This return of the P_{CO_2} to normal will cause the pH to rise again, and to a first approximation:

$$pH = 6.1 + \log\frac{23}{1.2} = 6.1 + \log 19.17 = 7.38$$

The body can do rather better than this as far as restoring pH is concerned, since the remaining fall in pH will stimulate the respiration. The alveolar ventilation will, therefore, increase rather than remain constant, and the composition of the alveolar air will move a little nearer to that of atmosphere air, so that the P_{CO_2} will drop a little. This will further increase the bicarbonate/carbon dioxide ratio and so the pH will increase a little further towards 7.4, so that the final position will be something like:

$$pH = pk + \log \frac{23}{1.16}$$

$$= 7.39.$$

A complete return to the normal pH requires other mechanisms, since a small fall in pH is required to maintain the increased rate of alveolar ventilation so as to maintain the lower than normal P_{CO_2} (at least in the short term). The end result shows that the acid is effectively buffered but that the bicarbonate concentration has dropped by an amount equivalent to the quantity of acid added. This was converted to carbonic acid in the initial buffering and lost as carbon dioxide. In practice, of course, these three phases of the buffering do not take place in succession, but all are continuing together all the time acid is being added. However, it is easier to visualize the contribution of the different components to the overall buffering by considering them one at a time. Thus, whatever the efficiency of the actual chemical buffering done by the bicarbonate system, the interaction of the chemical buffering with the 'physiological buffering' carried out as a result of the respiratory system controlling the P_{CO_2}, makes the overall system extremely effective.

This illustration is, of course, highly simplified as the plasma and extracellular fluid (except for the cerebro-spinal fluid) contain buffers other than bicarbonate, and also contain cells which, as described later (Section 1.10), also contribute to the buffering. The other buffers contribute to the initial chemical buffering of the acid, combining with some of the added hydrogen ions, and so reducing the number of bicarbonate ions removed. However, the 'physiological' buffering (i.e. that buffering due to control of

the P_{CO_2}) involves the bicarbonate system only, so in the return of the pH towards normal, the other buffers release their hydrogen ions again, to be taken up by bicarbonate and converted to water and carbon dioxide which is excreted via the lungs. Thus even in the real plasma or extracellular fluid, physiological buffering of 1 mmol litre^{-1} of acid will involve the loss of only a little less than 1 mmol l^{-1} of bicarbonate. Some of the added hydrogen ions do remain combined with the other buffers as the final pH is a little lower than it was originally. In any case, the end result is a return to a nearly normal pH, but with a lowering of the [HCO$_3^-$] and, to a proportionally somewhat smaller extent, of the P_{CO_2}.

In order to restore the plasma and extracellular fluid to its normal state, it is necessary to replace the bicarbonate ions which have been lost. Metabolic carbon dioxide can provide an effectively inexhaustible supply of bicarbonate ions:

$$CO_2 + H_2O \rightleftharpoons H_2CO_3 \rightleftharpoons H^+ + HCO_3^-$$

but since the generation of a bicarbonate ion is always associated with the generation of a hydrogen ion, the normal pH and [HCO$_3^-$] can only be restored if the hydrogen ion is removed in some way. Buffering cannot help since, apart from anything else, the removal of hydrogen ions by buffers is always associated with some rise in the 'free' hydrogen ion concentration. In fact, such removal of hydrogen ions from solution in the body fluids takes place only via the kidneys, where hydrogen ions are produced from CO_2 (and water) and secreted into the urine, while the simultaneously produced bicarbonate ion enters the extracellular fluid. This is dealt with more fully elsewhere (see Section 3.4).

To summarize these changes, acid added to the extracellular fluid is first buffered chemically, then 'physiologically', leading to the pH being restored nearly to normal. The bicarbonate concentration is now reduced and the P_{CO_2} is reduced because the alveolar ventilation is maintained at a somewhat increased level as a result of the slightly lower pH. Over the course of hours or days (depending on the quantity of acid involved), the bicarbonate concentration and hence the pH, respiratory rate and P_{CO_2}

will be restored to normal as a result of excretion by the kidneys of the same number of hydrogen ions as were originally added.

If alkali is added, the converse changes occur, with the chemical and physiological buffering leading to a higher than normal bicarbonate concentration, some depression of respiration and hence a higher than normal P_{CO_2}. Hydroxyl ions are excreted by the kidneys (in combination with carbon dioxide — as bicarbonate ions), as a result of bicarbonate ions not being reabsorbed from the tubular fluid, so that the normal bicarbonate etc. levels in the plasma are restored. The 'respiratory buffering' is less effective for large quantities of alkali than for acid since the reduction of the rate of alveolar ventilation which is necessary to cause a rise in the alveolar P_{CO_2} also causes a reduction in the alveolar P_{O_2} and hence in the oxygen saturation of the blood. Any large lowering of the oxygen saturation will tend to stimulate the respiration and counteract the depressing effect produced by the raising of the pH. Thus, the final compromise between these two effects will tend to leave the P_{CO_2} nearer to normal than it would have been for a comparable change in the acid direction, and thus leave the pH further from the normal value. In practice, this is not of much significance, since changes in metabolism which produce large changes in acid-base equilibrium, tend to shift the equilibrium in the acid direction rather than in the alkaline direction (see also Section 3.5).

The above account of the role of the bicarbonate buffer system in the plasma and extracellular fluid does not, of course, take into account what happens in the cells during or following a change in the pH. When the extracellular fluid pH changes the intracellular pH will change in the same direction (see Section 1.10). This means that following addition of acids, hydrogen ions will enter the cells (and potassium ions will leave) and there mostly combine with proteins and other buffers (principally phosphate). The effect is roughly that of providing additional buffers for the extracellular fluid, but with a relatively slow response time, since equilibration of the intracellular and extracellular pH seems to take a matter of hours. In the case of the red blood cells, not only do hydrogen ions enter the cells, but

bicarbonate ions leave (in exchange for chloride ions) providing additional buffering for the plasma. These movements take place quickly, since the red cell membrane (unlike most other cell membranes) is freely permeable to bicarbonate ions. (This provides the basis for the so-called 'chloride shift', the name given to the movement of chloride ions from the venous plasma into the red cells, in exchange for bicarbonate ions which helps to buffer the carbonic acid taken up from the tissues).

The mineral crystals in bone are also in equilibrium with the hydrogen ion concentration of the extracellular fluid. A rise in hydrogen ion concentration leads to an increased number of hydrogen ions entering the crystals in exchange for sodium or calcium ions. This process takes a considerable time to come to equilibrium. The bones thus provide additional buffering capacity for the extracellular fluid, again with a slow response time.

1.8 *Passive Membrane Properties and the Extracellular Fluid*

Animals contain a large number of different membranes separating various solutions from one another. For example, each cell membrane separates the intracellular fluid of its own cell from the extracellular fluid, and in the great majority of the tissues, the capillary basement membrane separates the plasma from the extracellular fluid. One property that most of these membranes share is that they are not uniformly permeable to all the substances in the solutions on either side and can therefore be described as being semi-permeable. In all cases where the membrane is permeable to any of the constituents on either side, these constituents will diffuse through the membrane. The composition of the fluids on the two sides of the membrane will tend to come into an equilibrium (although the compositions will usually not be identical unless the membrane is permeable to all the substances in the fluids). At this point, the passage of each substance through the membrane in one direction is at the same rate as its passage in the other direction. For some membranes, this equilibrium is purely passive, i.e. does not depend on any energy-

requiring (or active) process operating across the membrane (e.g. capillary basement membranes) but for others it does depend on processes which need a supply of energy (e.g. cell membranes).

The first case to consider is when two solutions of the same substance which are of different concentrations are separated by a membrane which is permeable to the solvent, but not to the solute. In the course of their random thermal movements, molecules both of solvent and solute will collide with both sides of the membrane, and some of the solvent molecules will pass through, a process usually referred to as diffusion. The solution with a higher concentration of solute has, in effect, a lower concentration of solvent, so that more solvent molecules will hit the side of the membrane on which the less concentrated solution lies. This means that more solvent molecules will pass through the membrane towards the more concentrated solution than will pass in the opposite direction. There will therefore be a net diffusion of solvent from the less concentrated to the more concentrated solution. This process will continue unless the rates of diffusion become equal. This may occur if sufficient solvent passes through the membrane to make the concentrations on the two sides equal. The rates may also become equal as a result of a difference in hydrostatic pressure across the membrane. A higher hydrostatic pressure on one side will tend to force solvent molecules through the membrane, and, at a particular difference of pressure, the (net) rate at which solvent molecules pass through due to the pressure will be equal to the (net) diffusion due to the difference in concentration between the two solutions. The pressure necessary to stop net movement of solvent through the membrane is equal to the difference in osmotic pressure between the two solutions. The osmotic pressure of a solution is the pressure needed to prevent net diffusion of solvent when there is pure solvent on one side of the membrane, and depends on the concentration in the solution of solute particles which cannot pass through the membrane. The osmotic pressures produced by different substances in a solution are additive, so that the total osmotic pressure depends on the total concentration of all the solute particles and will be referred to as the 'particle concentration' or the 'osmotic concentration' of the solution.

A molar solution of a non-ionized solute (e.g. glucose) has a total particle concentration of 1 mol l^{-1}, but a molar solution of, for example, sodium chloride has a total particle concentration of 2 mol l^{-1}, because it dissociates in solution into twice as many particles as does the glucose. The osmotic pressure produced is actually slightly less than twice that for glucose because the negatively charged chloride ions and positively charged sodium ions attract one another electrostatically, which somewhat reduces their contribution to the osmotic pressure.

In solution, molecules or particles of solute are in random thermal motion and so behave in some respects as though they were molecules of a gas. A substance in solution tends to expand, like a gas, and the osmotic pressure can be thought of as the pressure which has to be applied to stop it expanding, in the same way that pressure has to be applied to a real gas to stop it expanding.

From the physical laws for gases, for a gram-molecule of any gas:

$$PV = RT$$

(where P is the pressure, V the volume, R the universal gas constant and T the absolute temperature). At STP (0 °C and 760 mmHg or 1 atmosphere pressure) a gram-molecule of a gas occupies 22.4 litres, so, when compressed to occupy 1 litre, it will exert a pressure of 22.4 atmospheres. A 1 molar solution of a non-ionized substance also contains 1 mole of the substance in 1 litre, and on this basis should exert an osmotic pressure of (approximately) 22.4 atmospheres. This then is the osmotic pressure which a solution with an osmotic concentration of 1 mol l^{-1} should have. (Except in very dilute solutions, observed osmotic pressures differ quite markedly from the values calculated on this basis, since the interactions between solute molecules are really somewhat different from those between real gas molecules. Nevertheless, the analogy is still quite useful. See also Chapter 5 of ref. 13). For substances which ionize in solution, the particle or osmotic concentration will be higher than the substance concentration, because of the greater number of solute particles. For substances which ionize fully into univalent ions, the number of particles and hence the osmotic concentration is (as mentioned above) very nearly twice

that expected from the molar concentration. For such a solution, the osmotic concentration is the sum of the concentrations of the individual ions, measured in equivalents per litre. For solutions of polyvalent ions, the osmotic pressure will be lower than this, since there is more than 1 equivalent per 'gram particle'. For example, for a solution of magnesium sulphate ($Mg^{++} + SO_4^{--}$) the osmotic concentration will be half the sum of the ionic concentrations in Eq litre^{-1} but will still be twice the molar concentration (1 mole of $MgSO_4$ splits in solution into 1 mole of magnesium ions and 1 mole of sulphate ions. Each mole is 2 equivalents, making a total of 4 Eq). For multivalent ions, e.g. protein at the pH of the plasma, there are many charges on each particle so the concentration in terms of mol is much less than it is in terms of mEq.

For plasma as a whole, the normal concentrations of constituents present in concentrations greater than about 1 millimolar are, in round figures:

Cations	mEq	mmol
Na^+	145	145
K^+	5	5
Ca^{++}	2	1
Mg^{++}	2	1
	154	152

Unionized Substances	mmol	
Urea	5	(varies)
Glucose	4.5	(varies)
	9.5	

Anions	mEq	mmol
Cl^-	103	103
HCO_3^-	24	24
Phosphate	2	c. 1.2 (at pH 7.4)
Sulphate	1	0.5
Organic acid	c. 5	c. 5 (most are univalent)
Protein	19	1.5
	154	134.2

Total mEq of electrolytes = 308
Total mmol = 295−300

Note that the total numbers of mEq of anions and cations must balance exactly to preserve electrical neutrality, while the numbers of mmol contributed by anions and cations need not balance.

Consider now two solutions containing sodium chloride in different concentrations, but having another solute added to make the total molar concentration in the two solutions the same (to avoid the complicating effect of a difference of osmotic pressure). If these solutions are separated by a (hypothetical) membrane which is permeable to sodium ions, but not to chloride ions or the other solute, then there will tend to be a net diffusion of sodium ions through the membrane from the solution with a higher concentration of sodium ions. Each sodium ion that diffuses, however, carries its positive charge with it, so that the side of the membrane with the weaker sodium chloride solution becomes positively charged relative to the other side. In this way, a potential will develop across the membrane which will tend to increase the rate at which the positively charged sodium ions diffuse towards the negatively charged side of the membrane. An equilibrium will be reached when the diffusion of sodium in one direction due to the concentration difference is equal to the diffusion of sodium ions in the other direction due to the potential gradient across the membrane. The potential gradient required to bring the rates of diffusion to equilibrium depends on the ratio of the concentrations on the two sides, and the actual value for a given concentration ratio may be calculated from the Nernst equation (for univalent ions).

$$E = \frac{RT}{F} \log_e \frac{[Na_1^+]}{[Na_2^+]}$$

(where E is the EMF, R is the gas constant, T is the absolute temperature and F is the Faraday, which represents the electric charge (in Coulombs) on 1 equivalent of an ion. The subscripts by the Na^+s represent the concentration in solution 1 and solution 2 respectively.) The important point to remember about this equation is that it shows that the potential increases with the logarithm of the concentration ratio. This means that doubling the ratio will always produce the same change of potential

(approx. 17 mV) whatever the actual concentrations.

Since some sodium ions have actually crossed the membrane in order to set up the potential gradient, there will be a slight excess of sodium ions over chloride ions on the side with the lower concentration of sodium chloride, and a slight excess of chloride ions over sodium ions on the other side. However, the number of ions which actually cross is extremely small, too small to be detectable by chemical methods. This means that for all practical purposes, except the setting up of membrane potentials, the ions which have passed through the membrane can be ignored, and the rule that the numbers of negative and positive charges on the ions in any solution must balance holds good, even though in this respect it is not strictly true.

This line of argument can of course be applied to the equilibrium across a membrane for any ion present in the solutions on either side, so that an equilibrium potential can be calculated for each ion. Obviously, there can only be one value of the membrane potential for any particular membrane at any one time, and this potential will tend to drive positively charged ions towards the negative side of the membrane and negatively charged ions in the opposite direction. For any ion, if the actual membrane potential differs from that ion's equilibrium potential, there will be a tendency for that ion to diffuse through the membrane in such a direction as to tend to bring the membrane potential to its own equilibrium value (or, which comes to the same thing, to bring its concentration ratio into equilibrium with the membrane potential). Thus in the above example, the equilibrium potential for chloride would be equal in magnitude to that for sodium (since the concentration ratios are the same), but of the opposite sign. However, diffusion would not take place, because the membrane was defined as not being permeable to chloride ions.

To take an example nearer to real life, consider the effects of the properties of the capillary basement membrane on the solutions which it divides. This membrane is permeable to all solutes and ions of low molecular weight, but not to those of high molecular weight, like the plasma proteins. If such a membrane separates 2 solutions of sodium chloride, to one of which sodium 'plasma

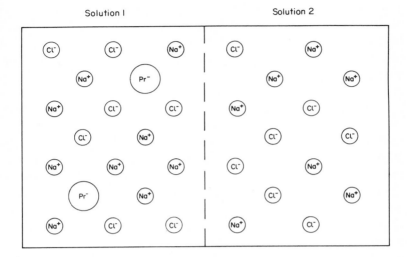

Figure 1. Diagrammatic representation of two solutions separated by a semi-permeable membrane. The protein ions (Pr^-) in Solution 1 are unable to pass through the membrane, while all other solutes can.

proteinate' has been added, then sodium and chloride ions will diffuse until an equilibrium is reached (see Fig. 1). The total numbers of positive and negative charges in each solution must balance. Thus, for solution 1 (measuring the concentrations in Eq rather than moles)

$$[Na_1^+] = [Cl_1^-] + [Pr^-],$$

while for solution 2,

$$[Na_2^+] = [Cl_2^-]$$

This means that if the sodium concentrations in the two solutions were the same, the chloride concentration would not be, and similarly if the chloride concentrations were the same, then the sodium concentrations would not be. If it is assumed that the initial chloride concentrations are the same (i.e. immediately after adding the sodium proteinate), then the sodium concentration of solution 1 will be higher than that of solution 2.

Sodium ions will diffuse into solution 2, tending to make it positive with respect to solution 1. This will make chloride ions follow the sodium ions, which (unlike the previous example) tends to cancel any potential difference between the two solutions. This means that diffusion will continue and a sufficient number of ions may pass to make a perceptible difference to the chemical composition of the solutions. Equilibrium will eventually be reached when the tendency for sodium ions to diffuse from solution 1 to solution 2 is balanced by a potential difference of appropriate size, with solution 1 negative with respect to solution 2. For this to be a true equilibrium with no net diffusion either of chloride ions or of sodium ions, this potential must also be equal to the equilibrium potential for chloride ions. There must, therefore, be a higher concentration of chloride ions in solution 2. This higher concentration is due to the chloride ions which have followed the sodium ions from solution 1.

Since the two equilibrium potentials are the same:

$$E_{Na} = E_{Cl}$$

$$\frac{RT}{F} \log_e \frac{[Na_1^+]}{[Na_2^+]} = - \frac{RT}{F} \log_e \frac{[Cl_1^-]}{[Cl_2^-]}$$

(the negative sign on the right-hand side is because the equilibrium potential for chloride is in the opposite sense since chloride ions are negatively charged). Cancelling, R, T and F on the two sides,

$$\log_e \frac{[Na_1^+]}{[Na_2^+]} = - \log_e \frac{[Cl_1^-]}{[Cl_2^-]}$$

Since $- \log (x) = \log (1/x)$, this equation can be written

$$\log_e \frac{[Na_1^+]}{[Na_2^+]} = \log_e \frac{[Cl_2^-]}{[Cl_1^-]}$$

Since their logarithms are the same, the ratios themselves must be the same, so that

$$\frac{[Na_1^+]}{[Na_2^+]} = \frac{[Cl_2^-]}{[Cl_1^-]}$$

or, multiplying both sides by $[Na_2^+]$ and $[Cl_1^-]$,

$$[Na_1^+][Cl_1^-] = [Na_2^+][Cl_2^-] \qquad (1.15)$$

(This relationship is a version of what is known as the Gibbs–Donnan rule. The Gibbs–Donnan rule proper is applicable to all ions, while this relationship applies only to univalent ions).

A corollary of this equilibrium is that where the concentrations on the two sides of the membrane differ, due to the presence of a non-diffusible ion on one side, then the total osmolar concentration of the diffusible ions is higher on the side with the non-diffusible ion. This can be shown quite easily.

In this example, let $[Na_1^+]$ be a, let $[Cl_1^-]$ be b and let $[Na_2^+]$ and $[Cl_2^-]$ (which are the same) be c.

Then, from the Gibbs–Donnan rule (equation (1.15))

$$ab = c^2 \qquad (1.16)$$

Now, in this example, a is greater than c and b is less than c. Let the difference between a and c be x. Then

$$a = c + x,$$

Substituting $(c + x)$ for a in equation (1.16)

$$(c + x)b = c^2 \qquad (1.17)$$

Now $c^2 > c^2 - x^2$ (for all real values of x except 0).
Substituting $(c + x)b$ (from equation (1.17)) for c^2 in this inequality

$$(c + x)b > c^2 - x^2.$$

Dividing both sides by $(c + x)$

$$b > c - x \text{ (since } (c + x)(c - x) = c^2 - x^2) \qquad (1.18)$$

The total concentration of the diffusible ions in solution 1 is $a + b$, and in solution 2 is $2c$. Now

$$a = c + x$$

Since, from equation (1.18), $b > c - x$,

$$a + b > c + x + c - x \text{ (unless } x \text{ is 0)}$$

$$\therefore \quad a + b > 2c$$

If the solutions in the previous example contain diffusible

ions other than sodium and chloride, these ions are all subjected to the same membrane potential and diffusion will therefore continue until the membrane potential is the same as the equilibrium potential for each of the ions. This means that all (univalent) cations will be distributed so that the ratios of their concentrations in the two solutions are the same and all (univalent) anions so that the ratios of their concentrations are the inverse of this. The ratio thus applies not only to individual ions but also to the total numbers of cations and of anions.

In plasma, most of the cations are sodium ions, and the majority of anions are either chloride, bicarbonate or protein. Considering a version of plasma, slightly simplified so as to include only these ions (in the round number concentrations given below), the value of the concentration ratios between the 'plasma' and 'extracellular' fluid for the diffusible ions is approximately 1.05, which corresponds to a membrane potential of about 1.3 mV, with the plasma negative to the extracellular fluid. The actual concentrations would be as follows (the concentrations in the extracellular fluid having been calculated from the values assumed for the plasma):

	Plasma (mEq)	Extracellular fluid (mEq)
Na^+	150.0	142.3
Cl^-	111.0	117.0
HCO_3^-	24.0	25.3
Protein	15.0	0

From these figures the total osmolar concentration of the 'extracellular' fluid is 284.6, while the osmolar concentration of sodium, chloride and bicarbonate in the 'plasma' is 285. The small difference in osmotic pressure resulting from this is obviously additional to the osmotic pressure due to the protein, which cannot pass through the membrane anyway. Thus there is a tendency for water to be drawn osmotically from the tissues into the capillaries as a result of the presence of the plasma proteins, both due to their own osmotic pressure and to the inequality of distribution of other ions across the membrane

which their presence causes. In the real tissues, although there is a great deal of diffusion of water and solutes, little net flow of water normally occurs because the mean capillary hydrostatic pressure just balances the 'colloid' osmotic pressure due to the protein. (There is, however, a net flow into the extracellular fluid at the arterial end of the capillaries, where the hydrostatic pressure exceeds the colloid osmotic pressure, and a net flow back again at the venous end).

1.9 *Cell Membranes and Intracellular Fluid*

The cell membrane is a semi-permeable membrane which separates the intracellular fluid of its own cell from the extracellular fluid. The extracellular fluid is of relatively constant composition from one tissue to another, but the properties of the cell membrane and the composition of the intracellular fluid differ from one type of cell to another. (In addition, the composition of the intracellular fluid may· differ from one part of an individual cell to another.) However, the cell membranes of the great majority of cells have a number of properties in common, and, partly as a result of these, the intracellular fluid in different types of cell is fairly similar in composition. In the following account some of these properties are described for an idealized representative cell, but it should be borne in mind that all features mentioned do not necessarily apply to all cells.

The cell membrane has a framework of a double layer of lipid material and also contains a good deal of protein. Substances which are soluble in lipids, such as carbon dioxide, can readily pass through the membrane. The membrane is also permeable to water and to many ions, although the permeability to different ions differs markedly. However, it is not at all permeable to protein. The intracellular fluid has an ionic composition strikingly different from that of the extracellular fluid. It has a much higher concentration of protein and of potassium and phosphate ions and a lower concentration of sodium and chloride ions than the extracellular fluid has. In addition, the inside of the cell is

negatively charged to a potential of about -70 mV relative to the extracellular fluid. Such a potential will tend to keep cations in the cell and keep anions out, so could, on that basis, be compatible with the observed potassium and chloride concentrations, but not with the sodium concentrations.

Most cells (under normal circumstances) have a constant volume and composition over a period of time, so that no net movement of ions into or out of the cell can be occurring. However, unlike the situation for the relationship between the plasma and the extracellular fluid, the cell is not in equilibrium with the extracellular fluid as far as the electro-chemical gradients of the various ions are concerned. This means that there will tend to be a net movement for each ion, in such a way as to make the membrane potential equal to the equilibrium potential for that ion. Such diffusion does indeed occur, and the constancy of the cell's composition can only be maintained by moving ions back against their electrochemical gradients at the same rate as that at which they are diffusing down. Moving ions against their electrochemical gradient is a process which requires energy and is thus an active process which depends on the metabolic activity of the cell. If the metabolic activity of a cell is stopped, e.g. by metabolic poisons, or by cooling, then over the course of a few hours, the composition of the intracellular fluid (and extracellular fluid) will change very much as the various ions continue to diffuse down their electrochemical gradients unopposed by the processes which move them back again.

The most important energy requiring process involved in the transport of ions through the cell membrane is the so-called sodium pump, which transports both sodium and potassium ions, the sodium ions out of the cell and the potassium ions into the cell. This mechanism appears to work in the same way in all types of cell, certainly all types of cell for which there are adequate data [44]. It has been estimated that somewhere between 10 and 20% of the metabolic energy of a cell is used by the sodium pump [27]. Although this is the main mechanism responsible for the long term maintenance of the difference between the intracellular fluid and the extracellular fluid, the passive diffusion

of ions is still governed by physico-chemical processes and what may be termed the passive properties of the cell membrane.

To provide an insight into the implications of this, first consider the passive properties of the cell membrane in relation to sodium and potassium ions only. Because of the concentration gradients, sodium ions will tend to diffuse into the cell and potassium ions will tend to diffuse out. If the potential across the membrane is to remain constant even in the short term, this diffusion must involve no net movement of charge, so that for each sodium ion that diffuses in, a potassium ion must diffuse out — i.e. the rates of diffusion of sodium and potassium ions must be the same. Since the ions are charged, their diffusion through the membrane forms an electric current, and the currents due to the two ions must be equal and opposite. The membrane offers some (electrical) resistance to this current and the resistance is different for sodium and potassium ions. The voltage driving the current for each ion is the difference between the actual potential across the membrane and the equilibrium potential for that ion. (At the equilibrium potential no net movement of the ion occurs, as described in Section 1.8).

The cell membrane is much more permeable to potassium ions than it is to sodium ions, which means that the (electrical) resistance to the flow of sodium ions through the membrane is much greater than the resistance to the flow of potassium ions. A much greater electrical force (i.e. voltage) is therefore necessary to drive a certain number of sodium ions (i.e. a certain current) through the membrane than is necessary to drive the same number of potassium ions through in unit time. Since the net electrical force for any ion depends on the difference between the membrane potential and the equilibrium potential for that ion, to make the sodium and potassium ion currents equal, the membrane potential must be much further away from the sodium equilibrium potential than it is from the potassium equilibrium potential. The precise membrane potential depends on the ratio of the permeabilities of the two ions, and the greater the sodium permeability in relation to the potassium permeability, the further the potential will lie from the potassium equilibrium potential.

The precise relationship can readily be derived, as shown in the Appendix.

It is difficult to accurately determine the concentration of ions in the intracellular fluid, but it has been estimated that the intracellular/extracellular ratio of potassium concentrations is about 15 : 1 and that for sodium ions is about 1 : 10. Taking these figures as correct, makes their equilibrium potentials −67.2 mV and +58.0 mV respectively (from the Nernst equation). The potassium permeability is at least 50 times that for sodium and is often much higher, so that the passive membrane potential would be −64.7 mV, on the basis of these approximate figures and a 50 : 1 permeability ratio (see Appendix, 2).

In order to maintain the cell in equilibrium in this condition, the sodium ions which diffuse in and the potassium ions which diffuse out must be transported back again by the sodium pump. If the sodium pump moved as many sodium ions out of the cell as potassium ions in, it would cause no net current through the membrane and so have no effect on the membrane potential. However, it appears that the sodium pump actually moves more sodium ions out of the cell than potassium ions into it, so that it creates a net outward current of positive ions through the membrane. This will tend to make the inside of the cell more negative, but the effect will be quite small and it is easy to work out what that the membrane potential will be at equilibrium if the ratio of sodium to potassium ion transport is known. It has been estimated that the pump transports 3 sodium ions for each 2 potassium ions (or some very similar ratio [44]). When the cell is in equilibrium there can be no net movement of the ions. This means that each type of ion is passively moving at the same rate (but in the opposite direction) as that at which it is being actively transported, so that 2 potassium ions are diffusing for each 3 sodium ions. Using the same argument as before, this means that the net electrical forces will be related to the permeabilities for the two ions in such a way that the sodium ion current is 1½ times the potassium ion current. This means that using the figures given in the above example, the actual membrane potential with the sodium pump active will be −65.6 mV, so that

the pump is only changing the membrane potential by 0.9 mV (see Appendix, 3). In cells whose membranes have a lower ratio of potassium to sodium permeability, the contribution of the pump to the equilibrium membrane potential will be greater since the (passive) membrane potential would be further from the potassium equilibrium potential (see Appendix, 4).

Although the situation for real cell membranes is rather more complicated than this, because there are other ions present to which the membrane is permeable, the ratio of sodium permeability to potassium permeability coupled with the different concentrations of these two ions is the main factor in determining the membrane potential. The membrane is also permeable to chloride ions, but in most cells these appear to be distributed passively across the membrane, i.e. their equilibrium potential is the same as the membrane potential. This means that no net diffusion of chloride ions occurs and the chloride ions have no effect on the membrane potential provided it remains constant (but will diffuse in such a way as to help to restore it, if it is altered). Other ions cannot pass through the membrane rapidly, either because of a very low permeability or because they are not present in sufficient concentrations. This means that the resulting current through the membrane will not have an effect on the membrane potential which is significant compared with that due to the currents of sodium and potassium ions.

1.10 *Hydrogen Ions and Cells*

The existence of the membrane potential does mean that all ions will tend to distribute themselves across the membrane so that their equilibrium potential is the same as the membrane potential, in other words, so that the cations are about 15 times as concentrated inside the cell and anions about 15 times as concentrated outside. In particular, this will apply to hydrogen ions, so that it might be expected that the intracellular hydrogen ion concentration would be about 15 times the extracellular hydrogen ion concentration. On the basis of a 15 to 1 ratio and an extracellular

concentration of 40×10^{-9} mol l^{-1} (or a pH of 7.4) the intra-cellular hydrogen ion concentration would be 600×10^{-9} mol l^{-1}, corresponding to a pH of 6.22. In fact, in the majority of mammalian cells for which pH measurements have been made, the pH is somewhere in the region of 6.8 [45], corresponding to a hydrogen ion concentration of 160×10^{-9} mol l^{-1} or only about 4 times the extracellular concentration and about one quarter of the expected value.

Since the cell membrane is very freely permeable to carbon dioxide, the carbon dioxide partial pressure in the intracellular fluid will only be a very little higher than that in the extracellular fluid even though the cell is continuously producing carbon dioxide. The bicarbonate concentration must be in equilibrium with the pH and the P_{CO_2} as represented by the Henderson—Hasselbalch equation (equation (1.13)). This means that the intracellular bicarbonate concentration must be about one quarter of that in the extracellular fluid or about 4 times the concentration expected if the bicarbonate concentrations were in equilibrium with the membrane potential. This situation can only be maintained either if the cell membrane is totally impermeable both to hydrogen ions and to bicarbonate ions or if there is some active process transporting hydrogen ions out of the cell or bicarbonate ions into the cell. The membranes of many cells (but not red blood cells) appear to be almost completely impermeable to bicarbonate ions but the permeability to hydrogen ions is probably similar to that for potassium ions (because the two types of ion are about the same size when hydrated). However, the concentration of hydrogen ions in the extracellular fluid is so low that the actual rate of diffusion of hydrogen ions into the cells is very small. (The equilibrium potential for hydrogen ions will be about -35 mV, so the potential tending to move them into the cell (about 30 mV) is smaller than that for sodium ions. Assuming that the permeability to hydrogen ions is comparable to that for potassium ions, i.e. 50 times that for sodium ions, the rate of diffusion of sodium ions will still be about 250000 times greater, since the sodium concentration in the extracellular fluid is so much higher —

150×10^{-3} mol l^{-1}, as against 40×10^{-9} mol l^{-1}, i.e. about 4 000 000 times greater). Even so, hydrogen ions must be ejected again at the same rate. The mechanism involved may well be related to the sodium pump, but the details are not known.

If the extracellular hydrogen ion concentration changes, the rate of diffusion of hydrogen ions into the cells will change in the same direction, so that the intracellular hydrogen ion concentration will tend to move as well. The cells however contain buffers, mostly in the form of protein and phosphate ions, in large concentrations, so that a small change in intracellular pH must involve the transfer of a large number of hydrogen ions into or out of combination with the buffer molecules. This means that if, for example, the concentration of hydrogen ions in the extracellular fluid falls, their rate of diffusion into the cells will fall. However, the cells will continue to (actively) extrude hydrogen ions at the same rate as before and this will now be higher than the rate at which they are diffusing in. These ions will help to restore the pH in the extra-cellular fluid. This movement of hydrogen ions will continue until the rate of diffusion balances the rate of extrusion, at a new equilibrium between the intracellular fluid pH and the extracellular fluid pH. The vast majority of these extruded hydrogen ions will have dissociated from buffer molecules within the cells as a result of the rise in intracellular pH. In this way, the cells provide a great deal of buffering capacity for the extracellular fluid, but it takes very much longer to act than the direct chemical buffering involving the extracellular fluid and plasma buffers. Dissociation of hydrogen ions from the intracellular buffers increases the number of negative charges on the buffer molecules inside the cell. For example:

$$H_2PO_4^- \rightleftharpoons HPO_4^{--} + H^+$$

In addition, as the pH rises, the bicarbonate concentration rises (since the P_{CO_2} remains constant) and this provides still more anionic charges. The cell membrane is impermeable to almost all of these anions so that as the hydrogen ions leave the cell, either other negative ions must leave or other positive ions must enter. Assume, in the first instance, that potassium ions enter the cell.

If many hydrogen ions leave the cell this is going to lead to changes in the concentration of potassium ions; a rise in the intracellular fluid and a proportionally larger fall in the extra-cellular fluid. This raises the ratio of the concentrations and hence raises the equilibrium potential for potassium, which in turn, as described above, will raise the membrane potential of the cell. This will lead to a redistribution of chloride ions so that chloride ions leave the cell tending to reduce the rise in membrane potential, but leading to a greater concentration ratio for chloride ions and so a new equilibrium at a higher membrane potential. This means that hydrogen ions leaving the cell lead to the cell having a higher membrane potential associated with a rise in the intracellular potassium concentration and a fall in the intra-cellular chloride concentration, with the reverse concentration changes occurring in the extracellular fluid. The change in the membrane potential also has some effect on the distribution of sodium and other ions [20].

Similar changes, but in the reverse directions, will take place following a rise in the hydrogen ion concentration in the extra-cellular fluid. The cells take up hydrogen ions, because the raised concentration in the extracellular fluid leads to a rate of inward diffusion greater than the rate of outward transport. Many of the hydrogen ions entering the cells are taken up by the intracellular buffers, thus slowing the fall in pH, which continues until the rate of outward transport again equals the rate of inward diffusion at a new equilibrium. This intake of hydrogen ions leads to a fall in the membrane potential and to loss of potassium ions and gain of chloride ions by the cell and there will tend to be a rise of the potassium concentration and a proportionally much smaller fall of the chloride concentration in the extracellular fluid. (The fall in the chloride concentration in the extracellular fluid will be much smaller in proportion than the rise of potassium concentration because, in changing the intracellular — extra-cellular ratios, approximately the same number of potassium ions leave the cells as chloride ions enter. This will be a very much smaller proportion of the extracellular chloride concentration than of the extracellular potassium concentration).

2. Renal Mechanisms

2.1 *The Role of the Kidneys*

The kidneys are the main excretory organs for the great majority of end products of metabolism, the main exception being carbon dioxide. The kidneys operate by producing a large volume of fluid (the glomerular filtrate), which has essentially the same composition as the plasma except that it does not contain substances of high molecular weight. The kidneys change the volume and composition of this fluid by selective reabsorption and secretion, and in this way change it into the urine which is excreted. There is thus no difficulty in excreting substances which are present in the plasma and which have a low molecular weight, it is only necessary to avoid reabsorbing them. This applies to many 'waste' substances, e.g. urea, but there are some low molecular weight substances which may get into the body and which cannot be removed in this way, either because they are taken up by the tissues so that none remains in the plasma or because they become attached to the plasma proteins and so do not pass into the glomerular filtrate. Such a substance is lead, and virtually no lead is excreted from the body once it has got in. This means that if inadvertent absorption of even very small amounts of lead continues over a period, the amount of lead in the body inevitably rises until it reaches an overtly toxic concentration. Some such substances may be removed from the body by injecting a substance of low molecular weight which does not combine with plasma protein and for which the substance has a higher affinity than it does for protein. If such a toxic substance forms a compound like this, it will be filtered into the renal tubules at the glomeruli and excreted (e.g. the

use of EDTA in lead and other heavy metal poisoning). However, such substances are outside the scope of this book, and, in general, only substances which are naturally present in the body will be discussed.

The kidney's most important task is to so adjust the final volume and composition of the urine that the body's composition, for water, salts, pH, etc., remains constant in the long term. The body's composition will only remain constant if the amount of each substance, or its metabolic precursors, entering the body (in food and drink) is the same as the amount leaving. Since urinary secretion continues throughout the day and night, while the intake of food and drink is discontinuous, there are bound to be short term fluctuations in the overall composition. For this reason it is most appropriate to think in terms of the input and output over a period of 24 hours.

The cells of all the tissues of the body are in contact with the local extracellular fluid. Since this has essentially the same composition as plasma, except that it contains much less protein, its composition is the same in all the tissues and forms the internal environment of the body. (This does not strictly apply to all tissues — in particular the central nervous system, where the extracellular fluid is cerebro-spinal fluid. This differs somewhat in composition from the extracellular fluid elsewhere. See Section 3.2). Any change in the composition of the body as a whole will, in general, be reflected by a change in the volume and/or composition of the extracellular fluid, so that if these are kept constant, the body's composition should remain constant.

The kidneys start their operations by producing a large volume of fluid, which has effectively the same composition as extracellular fluid, and modify this in such a way that what is reabsorbed and returned to the extracellular fluid maintains the constancy of the extracellular fluid; what is left over is excreted as urine. It is possible to infer the direction in which the kidneys are tending to change the composition of the extracellular fluid by comparing the composition of the urine with that of the plasma (or extracellular fluid — it is easier in practice to determine the composition of the plasma since samples of plasma are easier

to obtain than samples of extracellular fluid). If, for example, the urine is more concentrated (i.e. has a higher osmotic concentration) than the extracellular fluid, then the kidneys are tending to dilute the extracellular fluid.

Although healthy kidneys are capable, in most mammals, of so adjusting the urine as to cope with a wide range of intakes, they do have limitations (which differ in different species) which are a result of the ways in which the mechanisms for altering the volume and composition of the urine operate. For instance, in a healthy man the output of urine may vary between limits of about 300 ml and 16 litres per day, while maintaining the body composition constant. This means that if the overall net water intake (i.e. water ingested in drink and in food, plus water produced by metabolism, less water lost in breath, faeces and sweat) is less than 300 ml per day, the body content of water can no longer be maintained and it will drop. There are in fact three main areas in which the kidneys' capacity for adjustment may be insufficient to maintain a constant composition of the body: water, solutes and hydrogen ions — all of which are inter-related. The amount of water excreted is easily determined by measuring the volume of urine produced. As stated above, the maximum volume of urine which can be produced is about 16 litres per day. This limit is set by the glomerular filtration rate and the relatively constant reabsorptive activities of the proximal convoluted tubules (see Section 2.7); the urine will then be much less concentrated than plasma, because, under these circumstances, a much higher proportion of the solutes than of the water in the glomerular filtrate will have been reabsorbed. At the other end of the output scale, the urine will be concentrated, the maximum total osmotic concentration being about 4 − 5 times that of plasma. The limiting factor here is concentration rather than volume, so the minimum volume will therefore depend on the amount of solutes to be excreted per day.

The quantities of solutes excreted per day in the urine may vary quite widely, and for many substances the quantities vary independently. However, the quantities of ions which are excreted are constrained by the necessity for the urine to contain an equal

number of anions and cations. Most of the cations are either sodium or potassium ions and the minimum amount of these two ions combined which is excreted is set by the minimum number of anions in the urine. The number of sodium and potassium ions that are necessarily excreted in an alkaline urine is considerably greater than the number necessarily excreted in an acid urine, other things being equal. Thus, the pH of the urine may affect the total quantity of these two ions which has to be excreted (see Section 4.8).

2.2 *Renal Structure and Blood Supply*

The kidneys in an adult man weigh about 150 grams each, making about 0.4% of the total body weight; in different species of mammals they make up between about 0.2 and 1% of the body weight. The main bulk of the kidneys is made up of a large number of separate functional units which are called nephrons, of which each human kidney contains about 1 000 000. Each nephron consists of a tube closed at one end, and for descriptive purposes can be divided into four separate sections which are called the renal corpuscle, the proximal convoluted tubule, the loop of Henle and the distal convoluted tubule. The distal convoluted tubules of a number of nephrons join together to form tubes called collecting ducts which connect the nephrons to the ureters which convey the urine to the bladder (see Fig. 2).

If a kidney is cut in half lengthways, it can be seen with the naked eye that there are two clearly different types of kidney tissue, a layer of cortical tissue round the outside of the kidney, surrounding one or more areas of medullary tissue. This is shown on the diagram in Fig. 2. The cortical tissue contains the renal corpuscles and proximal and distal convoluted tubules of the nephrons, while the medullary tissue contains the loops of Henle and the collecting ducts. In some mammals, (e.g. the rat) there is only one area of medullary tissue in each kidney, while in others, including man, there are a number of areas each forming the centre of a separate lobe of the kidney. The urine formed in

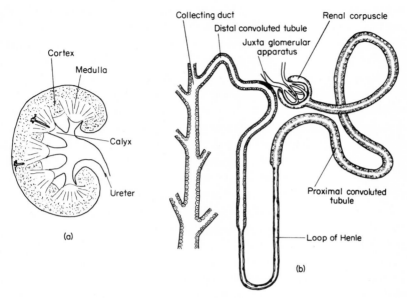

Figure 2. A. Diagrammatic longitudinal section through a multi-lobed kidney. The courses of a typical superficial nephron and a typical juxta-medullary nephron are shown to illustrate the differences in the lengths of their loops of Henle.
B. Diagram of a single nephron and its associated collecting duct system. See text for further details.

each lobe of the kidney enters a separate calyx of the ureter.

A renal corpuscle consists of a tuft of capillary loops, called the glomerulus, which is surrounded by a narrow space which is continuous with the lumen of the proximal convoluted tubule and which forms an expanded blind end for the nephron. This space is surrounded by a thin capsule called Bowman's Capsule. The remaining parts of the nephrons and the collecting ducts consist of tubes whose walls are formed by a single layer of cells (see Fig. 2). A proximal convoluted tubule winds around in the renal cortex near the corpuscle from which it arises before setting off towards the centre of the kidney where it becomes the so-called descending limb of the loop of Henle. The cells of the

proximal convoluted tubule have a very large number of fine processes extending into the lumen of the tubule which greatly increases the area of the membrane on this side of the cell. These fine processes make up what is called a brush border for the cells. The loops of Henle make hairpin bends and the ascending limbs are continuous with the distal convoluted tubules. Each distal convoluted tubule returns to the cortex to make contact with a structure called the juxta-glomerular apparatus. There is a juxta-glomerular apparatus related to each renal corpuscle, and a distal convoluted tubule makes contact with the one related to the renal corpuscle from which its nephron starts. The distal con-voluted tubule winds around in the cortex before joining a collecting duct. The collecting ducts successively join together as they run down through the renal medulla and finally convey the urine into a calyx of the ureter.

In all species of mammals, the form of the renal corpuscles and the relative lengths of the proximal and distal convoluted tubules are fairly similar. However, the lengths of the loops of Henle vary very much, both between species and, in many species, between one nephron and another. In man, and the majority of species, there is a wide range of loop lengths, those nephrons arising from corpuscles near the outer surface of the kidney having short or in some cases almost non-existent loops, while those arising from corpuscles lying deep in the cortex, close to the medulla (giving rise to the so-called juxta-medullary nephrons) have the longest loops (see Fig. 2), the maximum length differing in different species. In some species, on the other hand, especially those that live in arid environments (e.g. the kangaroo rat) all the nephrons have long loops of Henle. On the loops of Henle depends the ability to excrete a urine which has a higher osmotic concentration than plasma, and the maximum urinary osmotic concentration obtainable increases with the lengths of the loops of Henle. A major constituent of the renal medulla is the loops of Henle, and it has been found that, for a wide range of species of animals there is a very good correlation between the ratio of the thickness of the medullary and cortical tissue, and the maxi-mum urinary concentration which that species can produce [36].

The kidneys possess a unique internal arrangement of their blood supply. Blood reaches each kidney through a short large diameter artery (the renal artery) which arises directly from the abdominal aorta. For their size, the kidneys have a large quantity of blood passing through them — about 25% of the cardiac output when at rest (i.e. about 1¼ litres min^{-1} in an adult man). Nearly all the blood passes successively through two quite distinct capillary networks; first through the specialized high pressure capillary systems (the glomeruli) within the renal corpuscles, from which the blood leaves by arterioles (the efferent arterioles). These in turn lead to a second capillary network which closely resembles the capillary network in other tissues. The capillary networks within the renal corpuscles receive blood through short arterioles (the afferent arterioles) which branch off the terminal branches of the renal artery. These terminal branches run outwards through the renal cortex from vessels which lie near the junction between the cortex and medulla. Each afferent arteriole on its way to a glomerulus passes through the associated juxta-glomerular apparatus. This, amongst other things, appears to adjust the calibre of the afferent arteriole so as to regulate the pressure within the glomerular capillaries. The renal medulla has no direct blood supply of its own, but is supplied with blood which has already passed through the capillaries of glomeruli lying deep in the renal cortex, near the medulla — the juxta-medullary glomeruli. The blood passes down into the medulla and then back to the cortex through long straight capillaries which run parallel to the limbs of the loops of Henle. These capillaries are called the *vasa recta.*

2.3 *An Outline of the Functions of the Nephrons*

The different subdivisions of the nephrons have different functions. For descriptive purposes, each individual subdivision will be dealt with as though it were functionally homogeneous, although, certainly in the case of the proximal and distal convoluted tubules, this is not strictly true. In this chapter, a brief overall

outline will be given; each individual subdivision will be dealt with separately and in greater detail subsequently.

In the renal corpuscles, large volumes of fluid pass from the plasma in the glomerular capillaries into the Bowman's capsule by a process which is called ultrafiltration (see Section 2.7). This fluid is referred to as the glomerular filtrate and has a composition very similar to that of plasma, except that it contains none of the solid elements of the blood (i.e. red cells, etc.) and very little of solutes of molecular weight greater than 30 000 (i.e. the plasma proteins). The volume of glomerular filtrate produced is very much (of the order of 100 times) greater than that of the urine excreted in the same period of time. The glomerular filtrate passes on to the other subdivisions of the nephrons (where it is referred to as tubular fluid) and its volume and composition are greatly altered. In the proximal convoluted tubules, a large proportion of the solutes are reabsorbed together with an equivalent proportion of the water (so that the osmotic pressure of the fluid remains constant). This reabsorption continues at a relatively steady rate whatever the final volume and composition of the urine. In addition, a few substances are excreted into the tubular fluid from the extra-cellular fluid and therefore from the plasma in the capillaries around the tubules. The loops of Henle reabsorb some of the sodium chloride remaining in the tubular fluid, but very little of the water, so that the fluid leaving the loops of Henle actually has a lower osmotic pressure than the glomerular filtrate. This is at first sight rather surprising, as the function of the loops of Henle is to allow the secretion of urine which is hypertonic to plasma. However, the low osmotic concentration of the fluid is only a by-product of the loops' main activity, which is to set up and maintain an osmotic concentration gradient in the extracellular fluid of the renal medulla; the osmotic concentration rises towards the pelvis of the kidney. The ability to secrete a urine which has a higher osmotic concentration than plasma depends on this gradient.

The collecting ducts have in many respects similar functions to the distal convoluted tubules. In this part of the nephrons

further solutes are reabsorbed and some substances — notably potassium ions and hydrogen ions — are added to the tubular fluid. For most substances in the tubular fluid, particularly ions, the rate at which reabsorption and secretion take place can vary over a wide range. The reabsorption and secretion are normally regulated in such a way that the quantities of the various ions and water in the urine which is finally excreted, are such as to maintain the constancy of the body's internal environment, or to counteract any changes in the internal environment which may have occurred. The collecting ducts have one function which is not as such shared by the distal convoluted tubules. As they run through the renal medulla towards the pelvis of the kidney, they pass through the gradient of osmotic concentration set up by the loops of Henle. By adjusting the permeability to water of the walls of the collecting ducts, variable amounts of water are drawn out of the collecting ducts by the osmotic pressure difference between the fluid in the collecting ducts and the extracellular fluid. This allows the final volume (and hence osmotic concentration) of the urine to be adjusted.

2.4 *Renal Clearance*

In early physiological studies of renal function, it was found that, for a number of different substances, including urea, the quantity excreted in the urine in unit time was relatively constant, despite drinking large amounts of water to produce large changes in the rate of production of urine. In addition, for urea, it was found that if the plasma concentration changed, then the rate of its excretion in the urine changed in proportion [1]. Since the rate of excretion was directly proportional to the concentration of urea in the plasma, it appeared that the kidneys were removing the urea from a certain constant volume of plasma (or blood) per unit time and 'clearing' into the urine all the urea from this amount of plasma. This volume was termed the 'urea clearance' [32]. It was believed that this volume represented the volume of glomerular filtrate formed in unit time and that no urea

subsequently entered or left the renal tubules, so that this volume of plasma was actually cleared of urea.

It is now known that the urea clearance does not represent the glomerular filtration rate (see Section 2.5), so it does not represent a volume which is cleared of urea in the sense in which it was originally applied. It does however, still represent the volume of plasma which contains the quantity of urea which is excreted in unit time.

For any substance, the quantity excreted in the urine in unit time can readily be determined by measuring the volume of urine produced in unit time and the concentration of the substance. The quantity is given by their product,

Quantity (Q) = Concentration in the urine (U). Volume of urine (V) or, in symbols

$$Q = UV \tag{2.1}$$

The quantity of a substance which appears in the urine in unit time must be the same as the quantity removed by the kidneys from the plasma in unit time (unless it is a substance which the kidneys metabolise or synthesise). For urea, the quantity excreted in unit time is the quantity contained in the volume of plasma corresponding to the urea clearance. Thus

$$Q = \text{Clearance. Plasma concentration } (P) \tag{2.2}$$

Eliminating Q from equations (2.1) and (2.2),

$$UV = \text{Clearance. } P.$$

Rearranging this,

$$\text{Clearance} = \frac{UV}{P}, \tag{2.3}$$

It is obvious that the method summarized by equation (2.3) can be applied in the same sort of way to derive a value for the 'clearance' of any substance which is present in the urine and/or plasma. Experiments on substances other than urea have shown that different substances have widely different clearances, which in many cases alter considerably over a period of time, independently of the clearances for other substances. In addition, for

many substances, the clearance may change very markedly with changes in their plasma concentration. This makes the term clearance seem a misnomer, as the kidneys process the same plasma for all excreted substances and obviously do not process and 'clear' a quite separate and individually controlled sample of plasma for each different substance, but remove some of each substance from the whole of the plasma which passes through them. (There are however, a very few substances which the kidneys may more or less completely clear from the plasma of the blood passing through them). In spite of being in many ways inappropriate, the term clearance (or renal clearance) of a substance has remained in use for the volume per unit time which is calculated for the substance on the basis of equation (2.3). Even though (in most cases) such a figure does not represent a real volume of plasma which is actually cleared of the substance, it may nevertheless be of considerable practical use, as described in the next chapter.

2.5 *Use of Renal Clearances as Measures of Renal Function*

The regulatory activities of the kidneys are a result of the alterations which the tubules make to the composition of the glomerular filtrate in producing urine from it. The amount of regulation they are able to perform must therefore to some extent depend on the quantity of glomerular filtrate available to be modified. In many forms of renal disease, renal function is impaired as a result of loss of entire functional nephrons rather than of partial impairment of function in each nephron. For both of these reasons, an estimate of the rate of formation of glomerular filtrate gives some idea of the maximum capability of the kidneys for providing compensation for alterations of the internal environment, and comparison with the value for a normal but otherwise similar subject of the same species gives some idea of the degree of impairment of renal function which may exist. For healthy human adults and children of different sizes, the glomerular filtration rate varies with the surface area, although when

expressed in these terms it is somewhat lower for women than men. Very young babies, however, have an appreciably lower glomerular filtration rate than older children and adults and partly as a result of this have a relatively poorer ability to compensate for factors which tend to change their internal environments. For example, the maximum urinary concentration which a baby can produce is less than that for an adult and they are therefore much less tolerant of insufficient water or too much salt in their diet [35]. In renal disease, measurement of the glomerular filtration rate gives an estimate of the functional impairment of the kidneys whether due to renal disease, or to some other cause, e.g. dehydration or blood loss, both of which reduce the glomerular filtration rate and impair renal function as a result of a low arterial pressure and a reduced renal blood flow (see Section 2.7).

If any substance were present in the glomerular filtrate, and it was neither reabsorbed (actively or passively) from nor secreted into the renal tubules, then the rate of its excretion in the urine would be the same as its rate of entry into the glomerular filtrate. If the substance were unionized and of sufficiently low molecular weight to pass freely through the basement membrane of the glomerular capillaries, then its concentration in the glomerular filtrate would be the same as it was in the plasma. Thus the quantity of the substance entering the glomerular filtrate (in all the glomeruli) would be given by the product of its plasma concentration and the rate of formation of glomerular filtrate (usually referred to as the glomerular filtration rate or GFR). Thus (using the same notation as in the previous section)

$GFR \cdot$ Plasma concentration (P) = Quantity excreted (Q)

This is the same quantity as appears in the urine, so (from equation (2.1))

$GFR \cdot P$ = Concentration in urine $(U) \cdot$ Volume of urine (V)

from which

$$GFR = \frac{UV}{P}$$

By comparing this with equation (2.3) it can be seen that the glomerular filtration rate is equal to the renal clearance for such a substance.

Of the substances which have been studied, the one whose clearance is believed to give the best estimate of the glomerular filtration rate is the fructose polysaccharide inulin. This substance appears to be completely non-toxic, and its concentration in both plasma and urine is relatively easy to estimate. However, it is a substance which is not normally present in the plasma, so that to use it for determining the glomerular filtration rate it is necessary to infuse it intravenously at such a rate that its concentration in the plasma remains constant over the period during which its rate of appearance in the urine is measured. This makes the procedure rather complicated. For a number of species of animals, e.g. the dog, the creatinine clearance gives an estimate of glomerular filtration which is very nearly as good as that derived from inulin. Creatinine has the advantage of being naturally present in the plasma, since it is produced metabolically. Moreover, the rate of production is relatively constant so its concentration in the plasma remains constant (provided the glomerular filtration rate and hence the rate of excretion remains constant) at least for a sufficient length of time to determine its clearance accurately. In a number of species, including man, some of the creatinine which appears in the urine has, in fact, been added to the urine by secretion in the proximal tubules, so that the creatinine clearance is somewhat greater than the glomerular filtration rate. However, the amount of secretion is relatively small (see below) so that even in man the creatinine clearance gives a reasonable estimate of the glomerular filtration rate, and, equally important, an estimate of the glomerular filtration rate which is reasonably consistent in the same subject at different times and also between subjects. In addition, it is technically a great deal easier to determine the creatinine clearance than the inulin clearance, because the former does not need an intravenous infusion; this also makes it much more suitable for routine use.

It has been found that over a wide range of circumstances, the

urea clearance is consistently in the region of 60% of the glomerular filtration rate, as determined from the inulin or creatinine
clearance. For a normal human adult the glomerular filtration
rate is approximately 125 ml min^{-1}, and the urea clearance is
about 75 ml min^{-1}, or about 110 l d^{-1}, say 100 l d^{-1} in round
figures. The normal rate of urea excretion for a person on a
Western mixed diet is somewhere between 20 and 30 grams d^{-1}
(say 25 grams). It is possible to calculate the plasma concentration necessary to maintain this rate of excretion with a urea
clearance of 100 l d^{-1}:

$$\text{Clearance} = \frac{UV}{P} \quad \text{(equation (2.3))}$$

and

$$Q = UV \quad \text{(equation (2.1))}$$

so

$$100\,l = \frac{25\ \text{grams}}{P}$$

from which

$$P = \frac{25\ \text{grams}}{100\,l} = 0.25\ \text{g l}^{-1} \text{ or}$$
$$25\ \text{mg per 100 ml}$$
$$(4.17\ \text{mmol l}^{-1}).$$

The plasma urea concentration will be lower than this if the
rate of synthesis of urea (and the rate of excretion) is less than
25 g d^{-1}, as it will be on a low protein diet, and will be higher
if either the rate of synthesis of urea is increased or the urea
clearance is reduced (as a result of a fall in the glomerular
filtration rate). This means that, other things being equal, the
plasma urea concentration varies inversely with the glomerular
filtration rate, so that a value for the concentration may give a
rough estimate of the glomerular filtration rate. A reduced
glomerular filtration rate will nearly always be associated with
a raised plasma urea concentration, but a raised plasma urea does
not necessarily mean that there is anything wrong with the
kidneys themselves. It may reflect greatly increased production
of urea (perhaps from protein breakdown), or some extrarenal
cause of a reduced glomerular filtration rate.

For a substance like inulin, the renal clearance remains
constant over a very wide range of plasma concentrations, as

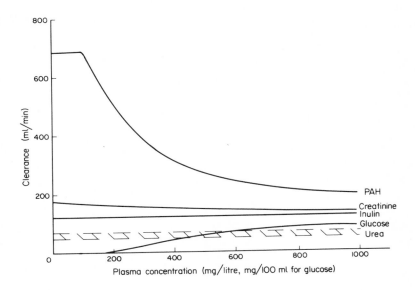

Figure 3. Clearance values for a number of substances at different plasma concentrations (for an adult man).

shown in Fig. 3. This is because the clearance depends only on the glomerular filtration rate, so, while this remains constant, the inulin clearance does also. The urea clearance also depends mainly on the glomerular filtration rate, and does not change as the urea concentration changes (but see below). For both these substances the rate of excretion in the urine is directly proportional to the plasma concentration. For many substances, however, the renal clearance does change with plasma concentration, and curves for a few substances which show a very consistent pattern are shown in Fig. 3. Since these are all substances of low molecular weight, their concentration in the glomerular filtrate will be the same as that in the plasma. This means that if the clearance is less than the inulin clearance, there must have been a net reabsorption of the substance from the tubular fluid between the glomeruli and the ureter, and, conversely, if the clearance is higher than that of inulin, then some more of the substance must have been secreted into the tubular fluid. Since some substances

are both reabsorbed and secreted, this only indicates which is the predominant process.

For two of the substances shown in Fig. 3, glucose and para-amino-hippuric acid (PAH), the clearance remains constant over part of the range shown, in each case at a level which is quite different from that for inulin. Over a considerable range, the clearance for glucose is 0. No glucose appears in the urine, unless the quantity of glucose in the glomerular filtrate of a nephron exceeds the reabsorptive capacity of that nephron. Above the level where all the nephrons are 'saturated', as the (constant) amount of glucose reabsorbed becomes a smaller proportion of the amount in the glomerular filtrate, the amount excreted becomes a larger proportion of the amount filtered, so that the glucose clearance approaches the inulin clearance as the plasma glucose concentration is increased.

For PAH, on the other hand, at low plasma concentrations, the clearance is constant and much higher than that for inulin, thus indicating that PAH is (actively) secreted into the tubular fluid. Experiments in which the concentrations of PAH in arterial blood and in renal vein blood have been measured have shown that over the range of arterial PAH concentrations where its clearance is constant, there is very little PAH in the plasma of the blood in the renal vein [41]. This means that almost all the plasma entering the kidneys is 'cleared' of PAH, so that the PAH clearance gives a very good estimate of the quantity of plasma flowing through the kidneys. Knowing the renal plasma flow, the renal blood flow can readily be calculated, provided the haematocrit (H) is known. The haematocrit gives the proportion of the blood which is occupied by cells, so that $(1 - H)$ is the proportion which is plasma. The blood volume is therefore related to the plasma value by the relationship

$$\text{Blood volume} = (\text{Plasma volume}) \frac{1}{(1 - H)}$$

so that:

$$\text{Blood flow} = (\text{Plasma flow}) \, 1/(1 - H)$$

and
$$\text{Renal blood flow} = (\text{PAH clearance})\, 1/(1-H)$$

This gives a reasonably simple indirect method for measuring the renal blood flow, which is a great deal more straightforward than measuring it directly. It does however, depend on the renal tubules being functional, and can only be used if the renal blood flow is reasonably constant over the period of measurement.

When the plasma concentration of PAH exceeds the level at which the clearance remains constant (see Fig. 3), the tubular cells are no longer able to transport all of the PAH in the plasma in the peritubular capillaries, so that some PAH is present in the venous plasma. As the plasma concentration increases above this level, the amount transported becomes a smaller proportion of the PAH in the plasma so that the clearance falls towards the clearance corresponding to the amount of PAH entering the tubules at the glomeruli, i.e. towards the glomerular filtration rate.

The creatinine clearance is consistently higher than the inulin clearance, showing that creatinine is transported into the tubular fluid by the tubule cells. As the creatinine concentration increases, the clearance approaches that for inulin, indicating that the higher the concentration, the smaller the proportion of the creatinine entering the kidneys which is transported. However, unlike PAH, creatinine does not show a constant clearance at very low plasma concentrations showing that the tubule cells cannot transport all the creatinine present in the plasma entering the kidneys however low the concentration.

For any substance, a renal clearance which changes with plasma concentration suggests that something other than purely physical (or passive) process is involved in its passage from the plasma to the urine. Urea has a clearance that changes very little with plasma concentration, and it is consistently lower than the inulin clearance. This suggests that no active processes are directly involved in urea secretion, but that some urea does passively diffuse from the tubular fluid. This is because the tubules are not completely impermeable to urea and the concentration is higher in the tubules than in the surrounding extracellular fluid. This is a

result of the reduction in volume of the tubular fluid as it passes along the tubules. However, it gives a less good estimate of the glomerular filtration rate than does the creatinine clearance, because the urea clearance does show some (inverse) variation with changes in the concentration of the urine [1]. The urea clearance is lower when the urine volume is low and its concentration is high; presumably more urea diffuses through the walls of the tubules under these circumstances, because the concentration gradient is steeper, at least in the distal convoluted tubules and collecting ducts.

2.6 Reabsorption and Secretion in the Kidneys

All the mechanisms by which the kidneys alter the volume and composition of the glomerular filtrate depend on their ability to move substances out of or, less frequently, into the tubular fluid. (Movement of a substance out of the tubules will be referred to as reabsorption and movement into the tubules as secretion). This reabsorption or secretion is defined as being either active or passive depending on whether or not, respectively, energy is required to move the substance. If the substance is travelling against an electrochemical or concentration gradient, its reabsorption (or secretion) must be active, while if it is travelling down a gradient its movement may be passive. In general, if passive reabsorption occurs, then active movement of some other substance must have occurred in order to set up the concentration gradient. (The reabsorption of sodium ions is quantitatively the most important active process involved). The movement of substances is effectively between the tubular fluid and the extracellular fluid around the tubules, and active movement — often referred to as active transport — always occurs as the result of the activity of the tubular cells and the substance travels through the cells, while passive movement may take place either through or between the tubular cells.

Active transport mechanisms in the kidney are classified as being of two types and are referred to either as rate limited or

as gradient-time limited mechanisms. (Although the differences between the two types of mechanism are not as fundamental as this implies, it is nevertheless quite a convenient sub-division in practice.) A rate limited transport mechanism (e.g. that for glucose) can transport the substance which it carries at a certain maximum rate. Provided the substance becomes available at less than this rate, all of it can be transported, but once the rate is exceeded, none of the excess is transported. This is thought to be due to there being a fixed amount of a carrier molecule with which the substance must combine in order to be transported through the tubular cell, and once this carrier is being fully utilized, no more of the substance can be transported. The maximum rate for such a mechanism is referred to as its Transport Maximum, commonly abbreviated to T_m. For many rate limited mechanisms, and certainly those which transport glucose and PAH, the maximum rate of transport is unaffected by the concentration gradient against which it is taking place.

Substances which are reabsorbed or secreted by rate limited mechanisms have characteristic ways in which their rate of excretion varies with their plasma concentration. This is shown for glucose and PAH, which are compared with the excretion of inulin in Fig. 4. This figure should be compared with Fig. 3 which is based on the same data, but presented in a different format. For inulin, the rate of excretion depends only on the quantity passing into the glomerular filtrate, which in turn depends only on its plasma concentration (so long as the glomerular filtration rate remains constant). For both glucose and PAH, above a certain plasma concentration, the graph becomes a straight line parallel to the line for inulin. The vertical distance from the line for inulin gives the rate at which the substance is being transported across the tubular walls. Where the graphs are parallel this distance is constant and it then represents the T_m for the substance (in mg min^{-1} in this instance).

At low plasma concentration, the glucose graph lies along the x axis since all the glucose is reabsorbed and none is excreted, while the graph for PAH is a straight line passing through the origin, but steeper than the graph for inulin. In fact, its slope

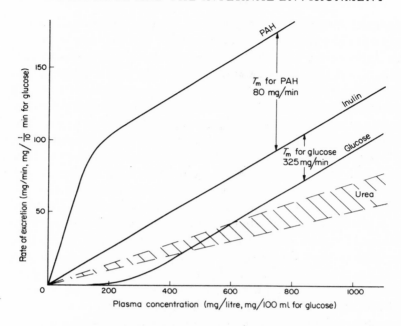

Figure 4. Rates of excretion of a number of substances at different plasma concentrations.

represents the PAH clearance in this range.

(For any point on a graph, the slope of the line joining the point to the origin is given by its y value divided by its x value. In this particular case the y value is the rate of excretion and the x value is the plasma concentration. Thus:

$$\text{Slope} = \frac{\text{Rate of excretion}}{\text{Plasma concentration } (P)}$$

or

$$\text{Slope} = \text{Urinary concentration } (U) \text{ Urinary volume } (V)/P$$

so that by comparison with equation (2.3) it can be seen that the slope of this line gives the clearance.)

A gradient-time limited transport mechanism (e.g. that for sodium ions or creatinine) is able to produce only a certain concentration or electrochemical gradient between the tubular fluid

and the extracellular fluid. It can only maintain this gradient if it has sufficient time, i.e. if the substance it transports is presented to it sufficiently slowly. If this rate is exceeded, the concentration gradient falls, although the actual quantity of the substance which is transported increases. The difference between this and a rate-limited mechanism in many cases, may be that the renal tubules are not totally impermeable to the substance being transported. This means that, as soon as a concentration (or electrochemical) gradient is set up by the transport mechanism, some of the substance starts to diffuse back down the gradient. Thus, the maximum gradient is reached when transport and diffusion occur at the same rate and then no net transport occurs. The balance between transport and diffusion obviously shifts towards the transport direction as the gradient falls, so that more net transport would occur, even at the same rate of actual active transport. Moreover, as the gradient falls, the energy needed to transport each ion or molecule also falls, so that more transport can take place for the same expenditure of energy.

The operations of the kidneys depend very much on the ability of the tubule cells to transport substances into or out of the tubular fluid. When a substance is unable to pass passively through the wall of the tubule, the cells may be able to transport the substance against a very high concentration gradient, but not at more than a certain maximum rate. If a substance is able to pass through the tubular wall, the cells are unable to set up a very high concentration gradient, and the rate of net transport will increase as the gradient decreases.

2.7 *The Renal Corpuscles*

In the renal corpuscles, the blood plasma in the glomerular capillaries is separated from the lumen of the renal tubules (i.e. Bowman's Capsule) only by a thin basement membrane. This membrane behaves as though it were perforated by numerous pores 7 — 10 nm in diameter, although there is no proof that actual pores exist. These 'pores' allow water and solutes of small

molecular weight up to $c.30\,000$ to pass through freely, while solutes of larger molecular weight pass through less readily. Any fluid which passes through the membrane from the plasma will contain low molecular weight solutes in (almost) the same concentration as in the plasma, but the substances of higher molecular weight will be reduced in amount relative to the plasma. For example, the concentration of albumen (molecular weight $69\,000$) is less than 1% of its concentration in the plasma. (In fact the anions and cations are not in the same concentrations, since the plasma proteins are negatively charged and do not pass through the membrane. Thus, from the Gibbs–Donnan rule, the concentrations of anions in the filtrate will be a little higher and that of cations a little lower than their concentrations in the plasma – see Section 1.8). The difference in concentration of the higher molecular weight substances means that there will be a lower osmotic concentration in the fluid in Bowman's capsule than in the plasma. Under normal circumstances the pressure in the glomerular capillaries is much greater than this osmotic concentration difference, hence fluid is forced out through the basement membrane into the Bowman's capsule in a manner analogous to pressure filtration – but through an ultra-fine filter – hence the term ultra-filtration. The rate at which fluid passes through the membrane will depend on the pressure driving it, which is the hydrostatic pressure difference across the membrane (i.e. the mean glomerular capillary pressure less the pressure within Bowman's capsule) less the mean osmotic pressure produced by the solutes to which the membrane is impermeable. (Since quite a significant fraction of the plasma volume passing into the glomerulus passes through the membrane, the large molecular weight solutes will be more concentrated and therefore exert a higher osmotic pressure in the plasma leaving the glomerulus than in the plasma entering it.) The proportion of the plasma entering the kidney which passes into the glomerular filtrate is known as the filtration fraction and may be estimated by measuring the ratio of the inulin and PAH clearances.

$$\text{Filtration fraction} = \frac{\text{Glomerular filtration rate}}{\text{Renal plasma flow}} = \frac{\text{Inulin clearance}}{\text{PAH clearance}}$$

Under normal circumstances in man, the afferent arterioles are of greater calibre than the efferent arterioles, so that their resistance to blood flow is much less, and the major part of the pressure drop between the renal arteries and the peritubular capillaries therefore occurs in the efferent arterioles. This means that the pressure at the afferent end of the glomerular capillaries is only a little below the mean pressure in the renal arteries and has been estimated to be about 70–80 mmHg.

What happens in the renal corpuscles under different circumstances can be described in terms of the glomerular filtration rate and the renal plasma (or blood) flow. Three variables may affect them, and these are the system arterial blood pressure, the calibre of the afferent arterioles and the calibre of the efferent arterioles. It is simplest to consider what may happen in a renal corpuscle when one of these changes while the others are kept constant, and only then to consider what may actually happen in practice.

The rate at which fluid passes out of the glomerular capillaries into the Bowman's capsule (i.e. the GFR) will increase directly with the pressure driving it. This pressure is the mean hydrostatic pressure (i.e. the mean pressure in the capillaries, less the pressure in Bowman's capsule which is small and will be ignored for the moment) less the mean osmotic concentration due to the substances which are unable to pass through the membrane. (The osmotic concentration of the high molecular weight substances will usually be somewhat higher at the efferent ends of the capillaries than at their afferent ends since an appreciable fraction of the fluid entering normally passes into Bowman's capsule.) Consider first what will happen when the systematic arterial pressure changes, but the calibres of the afferent and efferent arterioles remain constant. Blood flows through the afferent and efferent arterioles, so that there will be some drop of pressure across them which will increase directly with the flow which will in turn increase directly with the system arterial pressure. This means that the hydrostatic pressure in the glomerular capillaries will (to a first approximation) be a fixed fraction of the systemic arterial pressure. If systemic

arterial pressure is such that the glomerular capillary pressure is less than about 30 mmHg, no filtration will occur because of the osmotic pressure of the plasma proteins. As the pressure rises above this 'threshold', the rate of filtration will increase. It will increase in proportion with the difference between the actual pressure and the 'threshold' pressure, and hence more rapidly than the increase in total pressure (see Fig. 5). (For example,

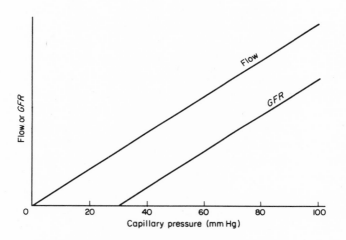

Figure 5. Relationship between glomerular capillary pressure and glomerular filtration rate (GFR) or blood flow. Note that the scales for GFR and flow will not be the same.

increasing the mean capillary pressure from 40 to 50 mmHg will double the filtration rate although it is only an increase of 25% in the total pressure. The effect is much smaller at higher pressures; increasing the pressure from 80 to 90 mmHg will increase the filtration rate by 1/5 ((80−30)/(90−30)) and the total pressure by 1/8). Since the filtration rate rises faster than

the pressure (with increase of pressure above the 'threshold') it also rises faster than the flow. Thus a rise (or fall) in pressure produces a proportional increase in blood flow, a somewhat greater than proportional increase (or decrease) in glomerular filtration rate and therefore some increase (or decrease) in the filtration fraction.

If the arterial blood pressure remains constant, changes in the calibre of either the afferent or the efferent arteriole will affect the renal corpuscle.

Constriction of the afferent arteriole will cause a rise in its resistance to flow, hence a rise in the total resistance to flow and a fall in blood flow. The pressure drop across the efferent arteriole will fall (because of the reduced flow across its constant resistance), so that the pressure within the glomerular capillaries will fall proportionately with the flow. (The pressure at the far end of the efferent arterioles from the glomeruli, i.e. in the cortical capillaries, being low and constant). Because the glomerular filtration rate falls in a greater proportion than the glomerular capillary pressure falls (see above), it will fall in a greater proportion than the blood flow, so that the filtration fraction will fall.

Constriction of the efferent arterioles alone will also cause a fall in blood flow, but some rise in glomerular capillary pressure (because of the reduced pressure drop across the resistance of the afferent arteriole). This will tend to increase the glomerular filtration rate slightly and hence increase the filtration fraction considerably, because of the reduced blood flow.

From the above it can be seen that it might be possible, by simultaneous alterations in the calibres of the afferent and efferent arterioles, for a change in blood flow to occur without any change of glomerular filtration rate or for a change in glomerular filtration rate to occur without any change in blood flow. Equally, changes in glomerular filtration rate or blood flow could take place independently of changes in the systemic arterial pressure, or, more important, blood flow and glomerular filtration rate could remain constant despite wide variations in systemic blood pressure. So long as the calibre of the afferent arteriole is

adjusted so that the pressure drop across it is equal to the difference between the actual arterial pressure and the required glomerular capillary pressure, then conditions within the renal corpuscles will not change. Obviously this can only apply when the systemic arterial pressure is higher than the required glomerular capillary pressure. The afferent arterioles do indeed appear to operate in this way to maintain a constant glomerular filtration rate and renal blood flow despite changes of systemic arterial pressure. The mechanism for this regulation does not depend on any neural control of the afferent arteriole and is known as auto-regulation. It has been suggested that alterations in systemic blood pressure produce purely physical changes in the pattern of blood flow, in particular the relative flow of red cells and plasma through the different glomeruli, and that this prevents changes in total blood flow or glomerular filtration rate although the rates in any individual glomerulus will change [33]. However, it seems more likely that autoregulation depends on appropriate adjustments of the calibre of the afferent arterioles and that this adjustment is one of the functions of the juxta-glomerular apparatus [40] (see also Section 4.3).

2.6 *The Proximal Convoluted Tubules*

The proximal tubules are responsible for the greater part of the reabsorptive functions of the kidneys. Almost all the normal constituents of the glomerular filtrate are reabsorbed to some extent; a number of them, such as glucose and the very small amount of protein that passes through the glomerular basement membrane normally being completely reabsorbed. Quantitatively the most important substances reabsorbed (in terms of numbers of molecules) are water, glucose and sodium, chloride and bicarbonate ions.

As well as possessing mechanisms for reabsorption, the cells of the proximal convoluted tubules are capable of secreting substances into the tubular fluid. Although there are mechanisms for transporting a number of substances, few of these occur

naturally in the body, the main one being creatinine. Although these mechanisms appear to have little function (some animals, e.g. dogs, manage perfectly well with tubules which cannot transport creatinine), they are of considerable practical use. The mechanism for transporting PAH makes it relatively simple to measure renal blood flow, as described above. The tubules are also able to secrete a number of substances which contain iodine and which are therefore relatively opaque to X-rays. This makes it possible to take satisfactory radiographs of the urinary system with injections of much less of the potentially toxic contrast medium than would otherwise be necessary.

The magnitude of the reabsorptive task of the proximal tubule can be calculated by comparing the amounts of substances which appear in the urine with those which pass into the glomerular filtrate. In a normal man, about 1.8 kg of glucose are filtered into the tubular fluid every day, of which none appears in the urine — all is reabsorbed in the proximal tubules. About 25 000 mEq of sodium ions and 5000 mEq of bicarbonate ions — or more than five times the total body content of each — are filtered and usually over 99% of each is actively reabsorbed, about 7/8 of this in the proximal tubules. Because so large a proportion of the filtered ions is reabsorbed, a very small change in the rate of reabsorption produces a very large change in the rate of excretion. For example, if the rate of sodium reabsorption falls by 0.5%, from 99.5 to 99.0%, then the rate of sodium excretion doubles. This large amount of active reabsorption requires a considerable amount of energy, and in man about $6-8\%$ of the resting energy consumption is used in this way. Since the kidneys are only 0.4% of the body weight, their metabolic rate is relatively high, although, as they receive 25% of the resting cardiac output, they extract a relatively small proportion of the available oxygen from the blood.

The pH of the tubular fluid as it passes down the proximal tubule remains fairly constant, and since the cell membranes of the tubular cells are freely permeable to CO_2, the concentration of bicarbonate must remain fairly constant as the volume of fluid diminishes. The tubular cells are relatively impermeable to bicarbonate ions, indeed if the tubular side of the cells were

permeable, bicarbonate ions would flow down their electrochemical gradient from the cells into the tubular fluid rather
than in the reverse direction (see Section 1.10). Unless the bicarbonate ions were removed from the tubular fluid, however,
their concentration would rise as the volume of fluid diminished,
and this would cause the pH to rise. They are in fact removed
in the form of carbon dioxide. The cells of the proximal tubules
actively transport hydrogen ions into the tubular fluid. These
are 'buffered' by the bicarbonate ions with the formation of
undissociated carbonic acid which breaks down into carbon
dioxide and water. This is perhaps not buffering in the strict
sense, since the added hydrogen ions produce no (or very little)
change in pH; the bicarbonate concentration does not change,
the total number of bicarbonate ions in the tubular fluid merely
decreases with the volume of fluid. The breakdown of the
carbonic acid to carbon dioxide and water within the tubules is
speeded up by carbonic anhydrase which is present in high concentration in the brush border of the tubule cells. This keeps
the P_{CO_2} and the concentrations of carbonic acid, bicarbonate
ions and hydrogen ions in equilibrium with each other.

The proximal tubules are freely permeable to water so that
as the various solutes are reabsorbed, water is also (passively)
reabsorbed and the tubular fluid remains throughout in osmotic
equilibrium with the extracellular fluid of the renal cortex and
hence with the plasma.

The reabsorption of sodium ions is the process requiring the
largest part of the kidney's energy consumption. It takes place
as a result of the activities of a sodium pump mechanism which
appears to be essentially similar to that which operates in other
cells (see Section 1.9). The sodium pump is probably also
responsible for the reabsorption of potassium ions. The active
reabsorption of cations from the tubular fluid creates a small
potential difference across the wall of the tubule so that the
tubular fluid is a few millivolts negative to the extracellular
fluid around it [8, 9]. This potential will of course tend to drive
chloride ions (and other anions) out of the tubular fluid and is
indeed the driving force for chloride ion reabsorption. The

inside of the tubular cells is at a potential of about -70 mV relative to the extracellular fluid, and therefore at a slightly lower potential relative to the tubular fluid. This potential is similar and also the potassium concentration within the cells is similar to that which occurs in many other cells. At first sight this suggests that the membranes on both the tubular side and the extracellular fluid side of the cells should be similar to those of the idealized cell described in Section 1.9, i.e. that they have a very much higher permeability to potassium than to sodium ions. However, there is a large net movement of sodium ions and a quantitatively smaller, but also important, movement of potassium ions from the tubular fluid to the extracellular fluid, so that the movements of ions across each membrane cannot balance. This means that the membranes cannot be considered in quite the same way as was used in Section 1.9.

On the side between the cell and the extracellular fluid there is a net outward flow of both sodium and potassium ions. There is no evidence to suggest that the internal composition of the cells differs markedly from the idealized cell considered earlier, so that sodium ions must be tending to diffuse in down their electrochemical gradient. The net outward movement of sodium ions would occur if the membrane were relatively impermeable to sodium ions and had a well-developed sodium pump mechanism (and a supply of sodium ions from elsewhere). The sodium pump would transport potassium ions inwards as well as sodium ions outwards, but a net outward flow of potassium ions would still occur if the actual membrane potential were removed far enough from the potassium equilibrium potential and/or the potassium conductance were sufficiently high to make potassium ions diffuse out faster than they were being pumped in. These things could happen with a membrane whose permeability to potassium ions was very much higher than its permeability to sodium ions.

At the membrane separating the cell from the tubular fluid, there is a net inward flow of both sodium and potassium ions. Since the fluid in the tubules is slightly negative with respect to the extracellular fluid, the membrane potential must be a little

lower than at the membrane on the other side of the cell and so even further from the potassium equilibrium potential (see Section 1.9). This means that there will be a greater electro-chemical gradient tending to make potassium ions flow out here than on the other side. In order to achieve net reabsorption of potassium ions, those ions originally present must be reabsorbed together with any which diffuse into the tubular fluid. The active transport of potassium ions into a cell is normally associated with the transport of rather more sodium ions out [44] (and there is no very good reason to suppose that the mechanism here is different), so the reabsorption of potassium ions is likely to increase the number of sodium ions to be reabsorbed. Sodium ions can enter the cells from the tubules by passive diffusion (since the electro-chemical gradient is in the right direction), and this provides the supply of sodium ions to be pumped out into the extracellular fluid on the other side of the cell. The total number of sodium ions which must diffuse into the cells is made up from the sodium ions which are reabsorbed plus any pumped out in exchange for potassium ions and any which diffuse back into the tubule from the extracellular fluid. The potassium ions comprise both the potassium ions originally present and those which have diffused from the cells into the tubules. The net re-absorption of sodium ions is very much greater than the net re-absorption of potassium ions, since there are many more sodium ions in the glomerular filtrate. This means that the number of sodium ions which diffuse from the tubules into the cells must be very much greater than the number of potassium ions which diffuse in the reverse direction. Since the potentials driving the currents of sodium and potassium ions are not very different from those for the idealized cell described in Section 1.9, this means that the ratio of potassium to sodium conductance for the membrane here must be very much less than for the mem-brane of the idealized cell, and also for the membrane on the side of the tubular cell separating it from the extracellular fluid. The walls of the proximal convoluted tubules are very permeable to both sodium and chloride ions [9]. Thus, a negative potential of the tubular fluid relative to the extracellular fluid will lead to

the diffusion of sodium ions into the tubule and chloride ions out of the tubule, so tending to neutralise the potential. The high permeability to sodium ions means that as soon as active transport of sodium ions out of the tubular fluid leads to the establishment of a concentration (and potential) gradient, sodium ions will start to diffuse back into the tubule. This means that it is impossible to establish a large concentration gradient but as the tubules normally operate against an extremely small gradient, few sodium ions diffuse back and a large number of sodium ions are transported. The large number of positive ions being actively transported out of the tubules creates the small potential difference between the tubular fluid and the extracellular fluid. This makes chloride ions flow out of the tubules at a rate sufficient to keep the total number of anions and cations leaving the tubule the same.

It is interesting and instructive to look quantitatively at some of the ion movements that occur in the proximal tubules. Although a great deal is not yet known about the details of the processes involved, the actual net quantities of ions which cross the tubule can be calculated. Making a few reasonable assumptions enables one to draw some tentative conclusions about some of the properties which the tubular cells must have.

Human proximal convoluted tubules are on average about 14 mm long and 60 μm in diameter [7]. This means that the surface area of a tubule is about $\pi(60/1000) \times 14$ mm^2 or about 2.5 mm^2. The total area of proximal tubular epithelium in the 2 kidneys is then about 2 000 000 times as much, making a total of about 5 000 000 mm^2 or 5 m^2. The tubular surface of the epithelium will be a little less than this and the extracellular fluid surface a little more. The glomerular filtration rate is about 180 l d^{-1} or 1 l every 8 min, and 4/5 of this is reabsorbed in the proximal convoluted tubules, so that 1 l is reabsorbed every 10 min. The sodium, potassium, chloride and bicarbonate ion concentrations of the tubular fluid do not change very much as the fluid passes along the tubules, so that the concentrations of these ions in the fluid that is reabsorbed must be similar to those in the glomerular filtrate and hence to those in the extracellular

fluid. Thus for each litre of fluid reabsorbed or about every 10 min, approximately 145 mEq of sodium ions, 5 mEq of potassium ions, 126 mEq of chloride ions and 24 mEq of bicarbonate ions must also be reabsorbed. The chloride ions are reabsorbed passively, probably mostly through the low resistance intercellular spaces [8, 9] while sodium and potassium ions are reabsorbed actively via the cells and bicarbonate ions are reabsorbed as a result of the secretion of an equivalent number of hydrogen ions into the tubules by the cells. These ionic movements are summarized in Fig. 6.

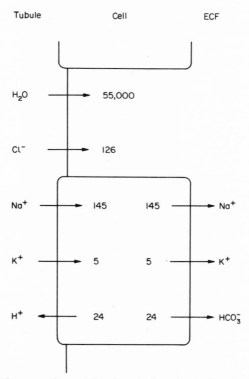

Figure 6. Diagram of a proximal convoluted tubule. The figures give the total net flow through all the proximal tubules of an adult man in mEq or mmol (10 min)$^{-1}$. (ECF = extracellular fluid).

There is normally very little difference in concentration between the extracellular fluid and the tubular fluid for either sodium or potassium ions. Although they are both being actively transported out of the tubules by the cells, there is probably little back diffusion through the intercellular spaces despite the small negative potential in the tubules, particularly as there is a large amount of water flowing out of the tubules (providing some 'solvent drag' (see p. 90 in [13]) outwards). Any such back diffusion will be ignored here, although any ions which do get back into the tubular fluid will have to be transported out again, so adding to the total transport by the cells.

At the membranes separating the tubular cells from the extracellular fluid, both potassium ions and bicarbonate ions will be able to move out of the cells down their electrochemical gradient, but sodium ions will have to be actively transported out. The actual number of sodium ions which must be transported is made up of those which have diffused into the cells on the tubule side (145 mEq per 10 min) together with those which have diffused into the cells from the extracellular fluid.

The surface area of the proximal convoluted tubules is about 5 m^2 or $5 \cdot 10^4$ cm^2. Because of the very complicated interdigitation of the cells of the proximal convoluted tubules [7], and the fact that the intercellular spaces are in continuity with the extracellular space around the tubule, the actual area of cell membrane involved is considerably in excess of this, perhaps 10 times as much, making an area of $5 \cdot 10^5$ cm^2. The passive permeability of cell membranes to sodium ions in those tissues in which it has been measured are quite low, and the rates of diffusion of sodium ions found have been around 10^{-11} Eq s^{-1} cm^{-2} [26]. On this basis, the passive diffusion of sodium ions into the extracellular fluid side of the cells will be about $5 \cdot 10^{-6}$ Eq s^{-1}, or 3 mEq (10 min)$^{-1}$ (This figure could well be out by an order of magnitude either way, but would still be considerably less than the number of sodium ions being removed from the tubular fluid). Thus the total number of sodium ions to be actively transported from the cells into the extracellular fluid will be 148 mEq (10 min)$^{-1}$ — say 150 mEq in round

numbers. The transport of these sodium ions outwards is almost certainly linked to the transport of potassium ions inwards, and if the 3 : 2 ratio found elsewhere applies here, then 100 mEq of potassium ions will be transported inwards. These together with those which have entered on the tubular sides of the cells must diffuse out of the cells down the electrochemical gradient for potassium ions. This makes a total of 105 mEq $(10 \text{ min})^{-1}$. The membrane potential is not very different from the potassium equilibrium potential, yet the rate of passive diffusion of potassium ions is, on this basis, about 30 times the rate of diffusion of sodium ions. If the rate of sodium diffusion has been guessed correctly, this suggests that the ratio of potassium to sodium permeabilities must be about 30 times higher than the ratio for the majority of cells (i.e. perhaps 2000 : 1), where the rates of diffusion of the two ions through the membranes are about the same.

At the membrane separating the insides of the tubule cells from the tubular fluid, the most striking feature is the large number of sodium ions which diffuse in. On the basis of the figures used above, it might be expected that only about $3 \cdot 10^{-5}$ Eq per 10 min would diffuse through an amount of cell membrane of the total surface area of the proximal convoluted tubules, or about 1/5000 of the actual rate $(150 \cdot 10^{-3}$ Eq per 10 min). However the area of the cell membrane on the tubular side of the cells is very much increased by the presence of the very large number of microvilli making up the brush border, so could be compatible with a sodium permeability similar to that of other cell membranes. If this is the explanation for the very high rate of diffusion of sodium ions, then it would be expected to lead to a similar increase in the rate of potassium diffusion (or in fact rather greater, because of the lower membrane potential on the tubule side of the cells). If this happened, the rate of potassium diffusion would also be of the order of 150 mEq per 10 min (or more), and 155 mEq per 10 min (or more) would have to be removed from the tubule. If this amount of potassium was reabsorbed in exchange for sodium ions on the usual 3 : 2 basis, this would transport 225 mEq of sodium ions

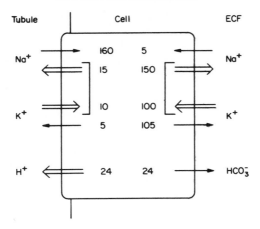

Figure 7. Breakdown of probable ionic movements through the proximal tubular cells (see text). Single arrows denote passive movements and double arrows denote active transport. Linked arrows denote linked ionic transport. Numbers as in Figure 6.

out again requiring a great deal of energy, and these sodium ions would have to diffuse passively back into the cells again. In fact, it seems that the permeability for sodium ions is not much less than that for potassium ions, as in the distal convoluted tubules [21] . (It is technically very difficult to measure the permeabilities of the membranes because of the high permeability of the tubular wall as a whole). If the permeabilities were similar, the rate of sodium diffusion would be much greater (say 30 times) than the rate of potassium diffusion, because the membrane potential is very much further from the sodium equilibrium potential than it is from the potassium equilibrium potential. On this basis, the rate of passive diffusion of potassium ions would be perhaps 5 mEq per 10 min, and in order to achieve the right net transport of ions, the overall ionic movements would be as summarized in Fig. 7.

In Section 1.10 it was suggested that the rate at which hydrogen ions diffused into cells was probably less than 1/250 000 of the rate at which sodium ions diffused in, so that the rate at which they were transported out was also 1/250 000 of the rate

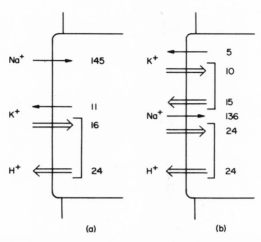

Figure 8. Ionic movements through the membranes separating the tubular cells from the tubular fluid. A. Assuming that hydrogen ions are exchanged for potassium ions. B. Assuming that hydrogen ions are exchanged for sodium ions. Symbols etc. as for Figure 7.

for sodium ions. In the cells of the proximal convoluted tubules, hydrogen ions are transported into the tubules at a rate which is very likely greater than sodium ions are, and which is only about 1/6 of the rate at which sodium ions are transported out of the cells into the extracellular fluid. The hydrogen ion transport mechanism is therefore very highly developed in these cells. It has been suggested that the hydrogen ions are secreted into the tubules in exchange either for sodium ions or for potassium ions. If they are secreted in exchange for potassium ions, it could be by a slightly modified sodium pump which transports hydrogen ions instead of sodium ions. In this case, they might be exchanged on a 3 : 2 ratio, as for sodium ions, which would give the overall ionic movements shown in Fig. 8A. If the hydrogen ions are exchanged for sodium ions, then this would reduce the number of sodium ions which have to passively diffuse in (although not by very much). If the exchange is on a 1 : 1 basis, then the over-all ionic movements would be as in Fig. 8B. In all of these 3 situations (Figs. 7, 8A and 8B) the rate at which sodium ions

diffuse through the membrane is much greater than the rate at
which potassium ions do.

From the discussion above, it seems very likely that the membranes on the extracellular fluid side of the cells of the proximal
convoluted tubules have very different permeabilities from the
membranes on the tubular side. The membrane on the extracellular
fluid side should have a very much higher permeability to potassium ions than to sodium ions, while that on the tubular side
should have permeabilities to the two ions which are not very
different.

2.9 *The Loops of Henle*

The loops of Henle, by active transport of sodium ions, act to
create a gradient in osmotic concentration within the medulla
of the kidney. Their arrangement as a long hairpin loop enables
them to produce a large overall range in osmotic concentration,
yet at no point are sodium ions transported against more than
a small fraction of this osmotic concentration difference. For
this reason the loops of Henle are often referred to as a 'hairpin
countercurrent osmotic multiplier' system.

The ability of the loops of Henle to set up and maintain a large
gradient of osmotic concentration through the renal medulla
depends on countercurrent systems. The properties of such
systems are perhaps easiest to visualize in terms of heat flow.
Consider first of all a heat-exchanger in which two streams of
water flow in parallel and at the same rate. If the hot water
entering is at 100 °C and the cold water at 0 °C, in the first part
of the exchanger there will be a difference of temperature of
100 °C so heat will flow rapidly. The temperatures of the two
streams will rapidly approach each other, but the 'cold' stream
can never reach a temperature above 50 °C and the 'hot' stream
can never get below 50 °C, however little resistance to heat flow
there is between the two streams (see Fig. 9A). If the direction
of flow in one of the streams is reversed, the situation is rather
different. The cold water entering receives heat from water that

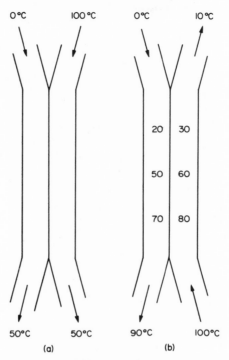

Figure 9. Heat exchangers. A. Parallel. B. Countercurrent.

has already been cooled further along the exchanger so the rate
of flow of heat and the rate of warming are initially less than
before. However the cold stream is always flowing towards
hotter water, so that heat continues to flow throughout the
length of the exchanger. At a particular rate of flow for a particular exchanger, there would be a difference of temperature
of 10 °C at all points. In this case, the initially hot water would
leave at 10 °C and the initially cold water at 90 °C (see Fig. 9B).
This 'countercurrent' heat-exchanger is thus much more efficient
in terms of transporting heat from the hot water to the cold than
the parallel flow one is. If the resistance to flow of heat between
the two streams is reduced (or if the rate of flow of water is
reduced, so that less heat needs to flow for the same temperature
change) the temperature difference between the two streams at
any point will be reduced so making the exchanger more efficient.

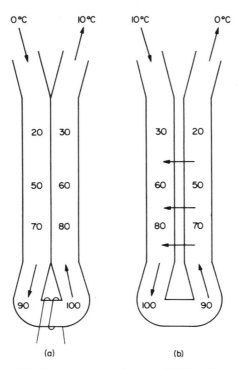

Figure 10. Countercurrent heat multipliers (see text).

Now consider a heater applied to a water pipe. If 10 calories (42 J) are applied for each ml of water which is flowing through, then a temperature rise of 10 °C will be produced. If the inlet and outlet of the heater are connected to a heat exchanger like that in Fig. 9B, to form the hairpin arrangement in Fig. 10A, then initially the water leaving the system will be only very slightly warmer than that entering, so that less heat is leaving than is being put in, and heat accumulates in the system. Heat will continue to be retained and the temperature to rise until all the heat being applied is leaving, i.e. when the water leaving is 10 °C hotter than that entering. When this state of affairs is reached the situation in the heat exchanger will be exactly as in Fig. 9B, so that the temperature of the water entering the 'hot' side of the exchanger will be at 100 °C. In this way the exchanger has acted as a 'countercurrent multiplier' and increased a temperature

difference of 10 °C across the heater (and across the exchanger at any one point) to a temperature difference of 100 °C between its ends. This illustration also shows up another property of countercurrent exchangers which is in effect to 'insulate' the ends from each other. In this case 90% of the heat in the water leaving the heater is returned to it, so that the temperature gradient can be maintained with only 10% of the heat which would be necessary without the exchanger. The insulating properties of heat exchangers are very important in the body. The flow of heat from the deep arteries to the deep veins of a cold limb allows the limb to receive an adequate blood supply without much cooling of the body core, since most of the heat in the arterial blood comes back in the venous blood and is not used to warm the limb, or, more important, the environment.

If the exchanger in Fig. 10A had a lower resistance to heat flow between the two streams, either the same gradient would be maintained for a smaller expenditure of energy, or a larger gradient could be maintained for the same expenditure of energy. In addition, the longer the heat exchanger is (provided the resistance to heat flow between the two streams remains the same), the greater the temperature difference between the ends per unit of heat put in.

Temperature gradients similar to those in Fig. 10A would be maintained if instead of heat being supplied by a heater at the tip of the 'hairpin', heat was transferred by some process from the ascending stream to the descending stream of the heat exchanger. If the rate of heat transfer was such as to maintain a 10 °C difference in temperature between the two streams at all levels, then the only difference from Fig. 10A would be that the ascending limb would now be colder instead of warmer, but the overall temperature difference between the ends would be the same (Fig. 10B). (To make the situation exactly the same, it is necessary to cool the water by 10 °C as it goes round the hairpin bend. It is also necessary to have the water entering at 10 °C instead of 0 °C. Apart from anything else it would freeze otherwise). Such an arrangement would then be very similar to the loops of Henle with the substitution of 'osmotic concentration'

for 'heat content'.

The action of the loops of Henle depends on the fact that the descending limbs of the loops are freely permeable to sodium (and chloride) ions and possibly water, while the ascending limbs are impermeable to water and actively transport sodium ions from the tubular fluid into the extracellular fluid, with chloride ions passively following due to the potential which this creates — as in the proximal convoluted tubules. The mechanism by which sodium ions are transported is probably the same as that which operates in the proximal convoluted tubules. However, here it is capable of moving sodium ions against a much larger gradient, because the passive permeability of the ascending limbs to sodium and chloride ions is very much less than that of the proximal convoluted tubules. At all points along the ascending limbs the osmotic concentration of the tubular fluid is of the order of 200 mmol l^{-1} less than that of the extracellular fluid surrounding them. At each point, however, the fluid in the descending limb rapidly equilibrates with the extracellular fluid because of the high permeability. Thus, at every level, sodium chloride will in effect be transported from the ascending limbs of the loops to the descending limbs, thus holding sodium chloride in the medulla in the same way as heat is held at the bottom of the system in Fig. 10B. In this way, the fluid in the descending limbs is continually increasing in osmotic concentration as it flows towards the tip of the papilla while that in the ascending limbs is continually falling in osmotic pressure as it flows back again towards the cortex. It can be seen that the concentration difference between the extracellular fluid in the renal cortex and the extracellular fluid surrounding the tips of the loops of Henle can be much greater than the concentration difference between the fluid in the ascending limb and the extracellular fluid at any one point. Also, the greater the length of the loops of Henle, the greater will be the concentration difference which they can produce. Continuous activity of the ascending limbs will be required to maintain this gradient, since it will tend to be dissipated by diffusion within the extracellular fluid, by the blood circulating through the medulla and also by entry of water from

the collecting ducts.

The blood supply of the renal medulla is from the vasa recta which run parallel to the limbs of the loops of Henle. This arrangement enables an adequate blood supply to be maintained with the minimum possible dissipation of the concentration gradient. As the blood flows down through the concentration gradient in the medulla it loses water and gains salts from the surrounding extracellular fluid so as to come to osmotic equilibrium with the surrounding extracellular fluid. Since the concentration of plasma albumen in the blood near the tip of the papilla is much increased, it appears that the movement of water is more important than the movement of salts [47]. If the blood then flowed out at the centre of the medulla, the salt which the loops of Henle were trying to accumulate there would be carried away but, as it is, the blood on reaching the depths of the medulla flows back again, giving up salt and gaining water again as it flows through the decreasing concentration of extracellular fluid. Since the blood (especially the red blood cells) does not instantaneously come to equilibrium with the extracellular fluid, the blood flowing down into the medulla will always have a slightly lower osmotic concentration (excluding the plasma proteins) than the extracellular fluid around the vessel, while that flowing back will have a slightly higher osmotic concentration. This means that some water is carried downwards and some salt upwards, tending to dissipate the gradient at a rate which depends on the rate of blood flow. Another result of the 'countercurrent exchange' in the vasa recta is that oxygen tends to diffuse from the descending to the ascending vessels and carbon dioxide in the reverse direction. This tends to keep oxygen out of the renal medulla and to keep CO_2 in, so that the P_{O_2} in the depths of the medulla is lower and the P_{CO_2} higher than in most tissues [29].

In the absence of any reabsorption of water from the collecting ducts, the maximum gradient which the loops can generate is limited by the rate of diffusion of sodium chloride and water within the extracellular fluid, together with their movement caused by the blood flowing through the vasa recta. However,

if some water is being reabsorbed, it will assist these processes
to dissipate the gradient, so that the overall concentration
difference will be reduced.

The more water that is reabsorbed the greater the effect it will
have, so that, for a given amount of work performed by the
ascending limbs of the loops of Henle, the less the maximum
concentration of the extracellular fluid near the tips of the loops.
Ultimately, for very large amounts of water reabsorbed, the
concentration will be only a little above that of the plasma.
Under conditions when water is being reabsorbed, both the distal
convoluted tubules and the collecting ducts are permeable to
water (see below). This means that the fluid entering the collecting
ducts in the cortex will be isotonic with the extracellular fluid
there, i.e. at an osmotic concentration of c. 300 mmol l^{-1}. In
producing a urine with a higher concentration than this, water
without any solutes must have been reabsorbed. The amount
of water which has been reabsorbed is readily calculated, if the
volume and osmotic concentration of the urine are known. This
enables the quantity of solutes in the urine (in terms of mmol)
to be calculated, and, from this, the volume of water that it
would have occupied at an osmotic concentration of 300 mmol l^{-1}.
(This quantity is ofter referred to as the 'osmolar clearance').
The difference between this volume and the volume of urine
actually secreted is the quantity of water which must have been
reabsorbed as the fluid passed down the collecting ducts. (The
fact that some solutes are also reabsorbed in the collecting ducts
makes no difference, since a corresponding quantity of water can
be reabsorbed with the solutes without any tendency to dissipate
the concentration gradient in the renal medulla).

To take a specific example, suppose the solutes in a day's
output of urine amount to 600 mmol of particles (which would
be a reasoanble figure for an adult man — Section 4.6), the maximum osmotic concentration of the urine will then be about
1200 mmol l^{-1}, so that the minimum urine volume would be
0.5 l d^{-1}. 600 mmol would however, occupy 2 l of solution at
300 mmol l^{-1}. Thus 1.5 l of water have been reabsorbed by the
collecting ducts during the day. If the quantity of solute particles

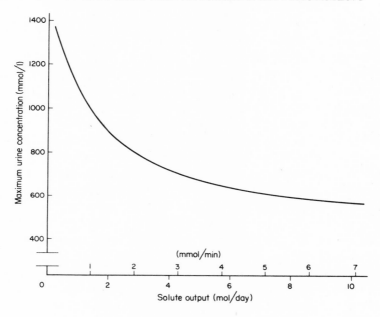

Figure 11. Maximum possible urinary concentration plotted against solute load for an adult man. From the data of Hervey *et al.* [22] and Rapoport *et al.* [34].

is doubled, to 1200 mmol d^{-1}, then this would occupy 4 litres of solution at a concentration of 300 mmol l^{-1}. In order to secrete this quantity of solutes in urine at a concentration of 1200 mmol l^{-1} (when it would occupy 1 litre), 3 l of water would have to be reabsorbed. This quantity of water entering the renal medulla would, however, reduce the maximum concentration. The 4 l of fluid at 300 mmol l^{-1} entering the collecting ducts would, in fact, leave them as urine at a concentration of about 1000 mmol l^{-1} and so would occupy 1.2 litres. Thus 2.8 litres of water would have been reabsorbed rather than 3 litres. Further increase of the quantity of solutes in the urine will lead to further reduction in the concentration gradient and thus further reduction of the concentration of the urine (see Fig. 11). Thus with a solute particle load of about 5000 mmol d^{-1} (which is really

only attainable under experimental conditions), the maximum concentration of the urine will be down to about 600 mmol l^{-1} so that the volume of urine will be about 8.3 litres. This means that 8.3 l of water will have been reabsorbed into the renal medulla from the collecting ducts.

2.10 *The Distal Convoluted Tubules and Collecting Ducts*

The distal convoluted tubules and collecting ducts share many of their functions and will therefore be described together. The fluid leaving the collecting ducts (i.e. the urine) varies very much in volume and composition from one time to another, but the fluid entering the distal tubules from the loops of Henle is relatively constant in volume and composition. This implies that the alterations of the tubular fluid which take place within the distal convoluted tubules and the collecting ducts must change from time to time. These parts of the nephrons possess mechanisms for transporting ions which are essentially similar to those present in the proximal convoluted tubules, but, unlike in the proximal tubules, the rates at which the mechanisms operate can vary over a wide range. It is this variability which allows alterations in the solute content of the urine, and the changes in the permeability to water of the distal convoluted tubules and collecting ducts (due to the effect on them of anti-diuretic hormone — see Section 2.12) which allows alterations of the volume of the urine.

The sodium reabsorption mechanism works in the same sort of way as in the proximal convoluted tubules; the membranes separating the tubular fluid from the interior of the tubular cells appear to be about equally permeable to both sodium and potassium ions [21], and since the (passive) permeability to ions of the tubules as a whole is very low (at least 100 times less than that of the proximal convoluted tubules [8]), the potential across this membrane is very much less than across the one separating the cell contents from the extracellular fluid. This means that the tubular contents are at a negative potential of

somewhere around 50 mV with respect to the extracellular fluid. This assists the reabsorption of chloride and other anions from the tubular fluid into the extracellular fluid, and the low membrane potential also increases the passive diffusion of potassium ions from the cells into the tubular fluid.

The mechanisms for secreting hydrogen ions into the tubules is well developed in both the distal tubules and the collecting ducts (especially the latter). While in the proximal tubules there is little difference in pH between the tubular contents and the extracellular fluid, in the distal tubules there may (in man) be a pH difference of 3 units (or 1000 : 1 ratio of hydrogen ion concentration). The proximal tubules secrete many hydrogen ions against a low gradient, while the distal tubules secrete a smaller number, but can secrete them against a much larger gradient. In the same way as in the proximal tubule, secretion of hydrogen ions can lead to the reabsorption of bicarbonate ions in the form of carbon dioxide. The pH finally reached in the urine will depend on the number of hydrogen ions secreted and the quantities of buffers present (see Section 3.4). Since the collecting ducts are permeable to CO_2 the final bicarbonate concentration of the urine will depend on the final pH (from the Henderson—Hasselbalch equation for bicarbonate, equation (1.13)).

The cells of the distal convoluted tubules and collecting ducts (and to some extent those of the proximal convoluted tubules) are able to synthesize ammonia from amino-acids, and do so mostly by removing the terminal amino group from glutamine or asparagine. E.g. (for glutamine):

$$COOH-CH-CH_2-C=O + H_2O \longrightarrow COOH-CH-CH_2-COOH + NH_3$$
$$\quad\quad | \quad\quad\quad | \quad\quad\quad\quad\quad\quad\quad\quad\quad |$$
$$\quad\quad NH_2 \quad\quad NH_2 \quad\quad\quad\quad\quad\quad\quad NH_2$$

The rate of synthesis is very variable and appears to follow the hydrogen ion concentration inside the tubular cells, but with a lag of 24 hours or so. If the acid-base equilibrium shifts in the acid direction, this increases the hydrogen ion concentration in the cells, so that they secrete more hydrogen ions into the tubules, and the rate of ammonia synthesis builds up over the next day or two. Equally, after a shift in equilibrium in the opposite

direction, the rate of ammonia synthesis falls off again over a day or two.

Ammonia is a base, since in solution it combines with hydrogen ions and so removes them from solution:

$$NH_3 + H^+ \rightleftharpoons NH_4^+ \qquad (2.4)$$

A Henderson—Hasselbalch equation can be written to describe the equilibrium for this reaction.

$$pH = pK + \log \frac{[NH_3]}{[NH_4^+]}$$

The value of pK is about 9.4, so that at a pH of 7.4 about 1 part in 100 of the ammonia will be in the form of NH_3 and at a pH of 4.4 only 1 part in 100 000 will be as NH_3 (and the remainder in both cases as NH_4^+). This means that a a pH of 7.4, 99% is in the form of NH_4^+, and at a pH of 4.4, 99.999% is as NH_4^+.

Ammonia (as NH_3) diffuses freely through the membranes of the renal tubular cells, while ammonium ions (as NH_4^+) do not (analogous to carbon dioxide and bicarbonate ions). This means that while the ammonia (NH_3) concentration will be much the same in the extracellular fluid around the renal tubules and in the tubular fluid, the ammonium (NH_4^+) concentration will be directly related to the hydrogen ion concentration.

The equilibrium for the reaction of equation (2.4) can be described by:

$$\frac{[NH_3][H^+]}{[NH_4^+]} = K$$

(where K is the equilibrium constant) so that multiplying by $[NH_4^+]$ and dividing by K,

$$[NH_4^+] = \frac{[H^+][NH_3]}{K}$$

This means that, given a constant ammonia concentration, the ammonium ion concentration is directly proportional to the hydrogen ion concentration. (The position is similar, but in the opposite sense, to that for bicarbonate, where given a constant CO_2 concentration (or P_{CO_2}), the bicarbonate concentration is

inversely proportional to the hydrogen ion concentration.) The proportion of 'total ammonia' (i.e. $NH_3 + NH_4^+$) which exists as ammonia (i.e. NH_3) is very small, both at the pH of the extracellular fluid (7.4) and that of an acid urine (< 7.4). This means that in an acid urine the 'total ammonia' concentration will be (very nearly) directly proportional to its hydrogen ion concentration.

The above gives the concentration in the tubular fluid and the extracellular fluid around the tubules which would be reached at equilibrium. However, strict equilibrium is not reached because the ammonia in the extracellular fluid is continually diffusing into the plasma of the blood in the capillary plexus around the tubules. This occurs because the ammonia concentration of the arterial blood will be much less than that in the extracellular fluid around the tubule cells which are synthesizing ammonia. Equally, the ammonia entering the tubules is being continually carried away by the flow of the tubular fluid. Although the ratio of the concentrations of total ammonia ($NH_3 + NH_4^+$) leaving the kidneys in the renal vein blood and in the urine will be near to the value which the equilibrium suggests, the ratio of the total quantities leaving by the two routes depends also on the ratio of the rates of flow of blood and urine.

2.11 *Hydrogen Ion Secretion by Renal Tubules*

The renal tubular cells, like almost all cells, are capable of actively transporting hydrogen ions outwards through their cell membranes. The mechanism appears to be much better developed on the tubular side of the cell than on the side next to the extracellular fluid. The cells of the proximal tubules seem to be capable of moving the hydrogen ions into the tubules against only a small gradient (between extracellular fluid and tubular fluid) but can move a relatively large number, while the distal tubular cells can move the hydrogen ions against a large gradient (of up to about 1000: 1 between extracellular fluid and tubular fluid) but in smaller numbers.

The transport of hydrogen ions out of these cells obviously tends to lower the hydrogen ion concentration within them. This tends to shift the equilibrium of the bicarbonate buffer system so that molecules of carbonic acid dissociate into hydrogen ions and bicarbonate ions. The carbonic acid concentration is maintained because the P_{CO_2} remains constant, since it is in equilibrium with the P_{CO_2} of the extracellular fluid and the cells contain sufficient carbonic anhydrase to maintain the system at its equilibrium position. The carbon dioxide concentration within the cells is maintained, not only because the permeability of the cell membrane keeps it in equilibrium with the P_{CO_2} of the extracellular fluid, but also, at least in the proximal tubules, for each hydrogen ion secreted into the tubule (and hence molecule of carbonic acid which has dissociated) a molecule of carbon dioxide diffuses out of the tubule, where it has been produced by the decomposition of a bicarbonate ion. Such processes within the cell can only continue in this way at a constant rate if the bicarbonate concentration remains constant. Thus the bicarbonate ions produced by the dissociation of carbonic acid within the cells must leave the cells, and in fact can readily do so by diffusing into the extracellular fluid down their electrochemical gradient. Since both hydrogen ions and bicarbonate ions are charged, in order to maintain electrical neutrality of the tubular fluid, the cell contents and the extracellular fluid, other ions must move at the same time. What appears to happen is that the hydrogen ion entering the tubular fluid leads to a sodium or potassium ion entering the cell. The bicarbonate ion can in effect accompany one of the sodium ions which is actively extruded from the cells into the extracellular fluid by the sodium pump mechanism and which is not balanced by one of the potassium ions simultaneously transported inwards.

The proximal tubular cells are known to have a membrane potential of about -70 mV, like most other cells, and if their intracellular pH and bicarbonate concentration are about 6.8 and $6-7$ mEq l^{-1} respectively (as they are for many of the mammalian cells for which these figures are known) then there is an electrochemical gradient for bicarbonate ions helping to remove them

from the cells. Presumably the membranes on the extracellular fluid side of the tubular cells are somewhat more permeable to bicarbonate ions than many cell membranes, since there must be a considerable flux of bicarbonate ions through them. (If the membranes on the tubular side of the cells were also permeable to bicarbonate ions they would diffuse into the tubular fluid, which would make the task of bicarbonate reabsorption more difficult).

Unlike the situation for bicarbonate ions, which can enter the extracellular fluid passively, hydrogen ions have to be move into the tubular fluid against an electrochemical gradient. The amount of energy needed to move a hydrogen ion from the cells into the tubular fluid obviously depends on the gradient. For a constant hydrogen ion concentration of the tubular fluid, as in the proximal convoluted tubule, the higher the intracellular hydrogen ion concentration, the less energy is needed (and vice versa). Factors which will raise the intracellular hydrogen ion concentration are a rise in hydrogen ion concentration (i.e. a fall in pH) or a rise in the P_{CO_2} of the extracellular fluid. This means that when both these parameters rise together, as occurs in 'respiratory acidosis' (see Section 3.3) the secretion of hydrogen ions into the renal tubules and hence the reabsorption of bicarbonate ions increases. On the other hand, in 'metabolic acidosis' when the hydrogen ion concentration rises but the P_{CO_2} falls as a result of the action of the respiratory compensation involved in 'physiological buffering' (see Section 1.7) there is a much smaller rise in hydrogen ion secretion for a given rise in hydrogen ion concentration in the extracellular fluid. This means that the rate of return to a normal pH and bicarbonate concentration is slowed. Thus the respiratory compensation for changes in extracellular fluid pH, although it is very effective in rapidly reducing the change in hydrogen ion concentration, actually retards the final return to normal conditions.

2.12 *Hormonal Control of the Kidneys*

Two hormones have very considerable effects on the activities of the kidneys in such a way as to be able to produce considerable changes in the volume or solute content of the urine. These are

antidiuretic hormone, which is secreted from the posterior lobe of the pituitary gland, and aldosterone, which is secreted (largely if not entirely) by the adrenal cortex.

Changes in the amount of circulating antidiuretic hormone affect the final volume of the urine without having much effect on the quantities of solutes it contains. Increased amounts of antidiuretic hormone produce a fall in the volume and a rise in the concentration of the urine. It has a number of actions which assist in the generation of a large concentration gradient in the renal medulla by the loops of Henle. The sodium transport mechanism of the ascending limbs is stimulated to some extent and the blood flow through the renal medulla is reduced. These actions both increase the concentration gradient, the first by stimulating the mechanism which produces it and the second by reducing its dissipation. In addition, in some species (certainly the rat and possibly man), antidiuretic hormone increases the blood flow and glomerular filtration rate in deep-lying renal corpuscles whose nephrons have long loops of Henle and reduces it in those with short loops. This increases the quantity of fluid passing through the loops which lie in the deeper parts of the medulla and so should assist in increasing the overall concentration gradient in the medulla. Antidiuretic hormone also increases the permeability of the distal convoluted tubules and collecting ducts to water. This allows the hypotonic fluid entering the distal convoluted tubules to come into osmotic equilibrium with the extracellular fluid of the renal cortex (by reabsorption of water). The fluid will also remain in equilibrium since water will be reabsorbed with the solutes which are re-absorbed during the passage along the distal convoluted tubule. As the fluid flows down the collecting ducts it will come towards osmotic equilibrium with the highly concentrated extracellular fluid at the centre of the renal medulla, before entering the ureters and the bladder which are impermeable to water. Even in the complete absence of circulating antidiuretic hormone there is a considerable concentration gradient in the renal medulla [5]. However, very little water leaves the distal convoluted tubules or the collecting ducts, and so the volume of urine excreted will be

only a little less than the volume of tubular fluid leaving the proximal convoluted tubules (i.e. about 1/8 of the glomerular filtration rate) and the osmolar concentration will be much lower than that of the fluid leaving the loops of Henle, because of the reabsorption of solutes which takes place in the distal tubules and collecting ducts.

The main effect of aldosterone is to alter the number of sodium ions which are excreted. In the process the quantities of a number of other ions in the urine are also altered. Aldosterone appears to act by increasing the permeability to sodium ions of the membrane on the tubular side of the cells of the distal convoluted tubules (and probably, but to a smaller extent, of the ascending limbs of the loops of Henle). This increases the rate at which sodium ions diffuse down their electrochemical gradient into the cells and hence increases the rate of reabsorption of sodium ions. This increase of sodium permeability will also somewhat lower the potential across this membrane (and hence increase the potential difference between the tubular fluid and the extracellular fluid) which will tend to increase the diffusion of potassium ions out of the cells into the tubular fluid. If the combined total of sodium and potassium ions (and other cations) in the tubular fluid is reduced to being only just sufficient to balance the charges on the non-reabsorbable anions, the reabsorption of a sodium ion leads necessarily to the excretion of another potassium ion (see Section 4.9). Thus the effect of an increased aldosterone concentration in the circulating blood will be to increase the reabsorption of sodium ions and hence decrease their excretion, and will also tend to increase the rate of potassium secretion.

3. Acid–Base Equilibrium

3.1 *Sources of Acid and Base in the Body*

Apart from the highly artificial situation where acid or base is injected intravenously, 'excess' acid or base usually tends to accumulate fairly slowly in the body. (This applies except in circumstances like severe muscular exercise or asphyxia where anaerobic metabolism leads to the rapid production of substances such as lactic acid in large quantities — see Section 3.5). Changes in the acid-base equilibrium of the body may be quantified in terms of the number of hydrogen (or hydroxyl) ions which have to be removed in order to maintain constant or return to normal the pH of the body fluids. Alterations in the equilibrium are usually a result of changes in the overall balance of metabolism, but may also occur if a fluid with a pH different from that of the extracellular fluid is lost from the body. The urine is such a fluid, but normally the pH of the urine is changed to compensate for alterations in the acid-base equilibrium of the body and its production does not normally cause the alterations. Loss of gastric juice will however cause an alteration in the equilibrium since it is highly acid, so that continued vomiting will lead to a tendency for the pH of the body fluids to rise. Indeed, the secretion of gastric juice following a meal produces a detectable, but short-lived rise in the plasma pH, the so-called alkaline tide (see Section 3.3).

In the normal course of metabolism large amounts of carbon dioxide are produced by the oxidative metabolism of organic compounds. The carbon dioxide enters the extracellular fluid from the cells and from here rapidly diffuses into the plasma in the capillaries, since the P_{CO_2} in the plasma is lower than that in the

extracellular fluid, where it is in turn lower than in the cells where CO_2 is produced. Carbon dioxide diffuses rapidly through aqueous solutions and also, being lipid soluble, passes rapidly through the membranes of most cells. From the plasma, the carbon dioxide diffuses into the red cells where it is rapidly hydrated due to the presence of carbonic anhydrase, which greatly accelerates the reaching of equilibrium in the first part of the reaction:

$$CO_2 + H_2O \rightleftharpoons H_2CO_3 \rightleftharpoons H^+ + HCO_3^-$$

(equilibrium being reached in the order of 0.3 s instead of the several minutes which it would take in the absence of carbonic anhydrase). The concentration of the carbonic acid equilibrates with the concentrations of hydrogen ions and bicarbonate ions almost instantaneously without any catalyst, and, because the haemoglobin simultaneously gives off oxygen, which changes the dissociation constants of its 'acidic' groups, the hydrogen ions are mostly taken up by haemoglobin with very little change in pH. Because the membrane of the red cells is permeable to bicarbonate ions they are able to enter the plasma (in exchange for chloride ions) thus increasing the $[HCO_3^-]$ nearly in proportion to the P_{CO_2}, again minimizing the change in pH. The reverse changes take place in the lungs, and the P_{CO_2} of the plasma comes into equilibrium with that of the alveolar air. This means that provided the rate of production of CO_2 and the alveolar ventilation remain constant, the movement of carbon dioxide from the cells to the outside air will continue steadily and there will be no tendency for the P_{CO_2} to change significantly at any point in the system. Thus although the P_{CO_2}, the pH and the bicarbonate concentration will differ somewhat in different compartments of the extracellular fluid (e.g. extracellular fluid, arterial plasma and venous plasma) and the values may differ in different tissues which have different rates of CO_2 production, in the steady state there is no tendency for any of the values to change. Although a very large amount of potential acid is produced (about 15000 mEq d^{-1} in an adult man) this does not (normally) give rise to any tendency for the pH of the body to

change. Although this applies to those substances which the majority of the tissues use as a direct source of energy (e.g. glucose, glycogen, etc.) and which are completely metabolized to carbon dioxide (which is effectively not acid, as described above) and water (which is neutral), it does not necessarily apply to those substances which are absorbed from the gastro-intestinal tract and which are the ultimate sources of metabolic energy for the body.

The actual content of acids and/or bases in the diet (and which are absorbed) will obviously tend to affect the pH of the body. However, this is not usually a major source of acids or bases, at least for mammals, since they eat mostly organic materials which are effectively more or less neutral as far as their actual pH is concerned. There are, however, two main classes of substances which are commonly present in the diet and which give rise to acid or basic end products (other than carbon dioxide) when they are metabolized. The salts of organic acids, present in large quantities in many fruits and other vegetable foods, produce basic end products, while proteins, particularly animal proteins, produce acid end products.

Salts of organic acids are basic because, in general, the un-dissociated form of the acid rather than the anion is completely metabolized. E.g. for citric acid:

$$C_3H_5(COOH)_3 + 5O_2 \longrightarrow 6CO_2 + 4H_2O$$

Citric acid itself is completely metabolized but a citrate or other organic ion (e.g. $C_3H_5(COOH)_2-COO^-$) can only be completely metabolized to carbon dioxide and water following combination with a hydrogen ion. Thus, metabolism of the ions effectively acts as a base since it leads to hydrogen ions being removed from solution. Proteins in the diet are acid mainly because they contain sulphur-containing amino-acids [25]. Other amino-acids are either incorporated into new protein or broken down to carbon dioxide, water and urea, all of which are effectively neutral. Each sulphur atom in the sulphur-containing amino-acids is oxidized to a sulphate ion, and this also involves the production of two

hydrogen ions:

$$S + 1\frac{1}{2}O_2 + H_2O \longrightarrow SO_4^{--} + 2H^+$$

The hydrogen ions have to be disposed of in some way in order for the pH of the body not to change. Since animal proteins are usually richer in sulphur containing amino acids than are vegetable proteins, animal proteins are more strongly acid producing. Thus, to maintain acid-base equilibrium on their normal diets, herbivores have to excrete an alkaline urine, while carnivores have to excrete an acid urine. On a mixed diet, the overall effect obviously depends on the relative amounts of acid-producing and base-producing substances in the diet. Man, at least on a normal Western mixed diet, consumes more acid-producing than base-producing substances. Thus, in order to maintain the pH of the extracellular fluid, the kidneys must produce a urine of a composition appropriate to remove the excess of acid.

For experimental (and for therapeutic) purposes, it is possible to alter the balance of metabolism by giving acids or bases by mouth or by giving substances whose metabolism produces acid or base. In order to alter the balance in an acid direction, ammonium chloride has often been used. This is a somewhat acid substance in solution because ammonium ions tend to dissociate into ammonia and hydrogen ions.

$$NH_4 \rightleftharpoons NH_3 + H^+$$

At the pH of the extracellular fluid, the equilibrium of this reaction is such that only about 1% of the ammonium ions are dissociated (see Section 2.9). However, on being absorbed from the gut, the ammonium ions pass to the liver, where ammonia is rapidly converted to urea:

$$2NH_3 + CO_2 \longrightarrow CO(NH_2) + H_2O$$

so that the ammonia (as NH_3) concentration tends to fall and some more ammonium ions dissociate, releasing hydrogen ions into solution. The end result is that a number of hydrogen ions equivalent to the number of ammonium ions absorbed have to be disposed of by the body. Another substance which has frequently been used to 'acidify' the metabolism is calcium

chloride. This substance is slightly acid because, in solution, calcium ions have a slightly greater affinity for hydroxyl ions than chloride ions have for hydrogen ions. However, its acidifying effect is not due to this, but to the fact that the calcium salts of most organic acids present in the diet (e.g. citrate) are insoluble at the pH which there is in the small intestine (something above 8) so that the organic anions are not absorbed. Calcium chloride thus acts by preventing absorption of base-producing substances and so altering the balance of metabolism in an acid direction, rather than by any direct acid-producing action. The substances which have commonly been used to move the metabolic balance in a basic direction are sodium bicarbonate, a base in its own right, and salts of organic acids, e.g. potassium citrate or sodium lactate, whose mode of action has already been described.

3.2 *The Cerebro-Spinal Fluid and the Control of Respiration*

Because of the way in which the carbonic acid − bicarbonate buffer system works, the pH of the extracellular fluid depends very much on the partial pressure of carbon dioxide (see Section 1.7). Short term regulation of the pH may indeed be achieved entirely by regulating the P_{CO_2}. The P_{CO_2} in the extracellular fluid depends on the P_{CO_2} of the alveolar air with which the blood comes into equilibrium as it passes through the lungs. The P_{CO_2} of the alveolar air depends in turn on the rate at which carbon dioxide is passing into it from the blood (which at equilibrium is the same as the rate of production of CO_2) and (inversely) on the rate at which the alveolar air is being replaced with fresh atmospheric air − the alveolar ventilation rate (see Section 1.7). It is therefore important to know some details of how the alveolar ventilation rate is controlled.

The extracellular fluid in the great majority of the tissues in the body comes very rapidly into equilibrium with changes in the plasma concentrations of all substances except those of high molecular weight (i.e. proteins). This is because the capillary basement membrane is freely permeable to low molecular weight

substances. However, the extracellular fluid for the central
nervous system, which is referred to as the cerebro-spinal fluid
(or CSF for short), differs in composition from the plasma and,
even for low molecular weight substances, a change in concentration in the plasma is usually followed only slowly by a corresponding change in the cerebro-spinal fluid, a new equilibrium
being reached only after many hours. Indeed, there are many
substances which do not pass from the plasma into the CSF at
all. The slowness with which equilibrium is reached and the
differences between plasma and CSF have given rise to the
concept of a 'blood-brain barrier' separating the plasma from the
CSF and central nervous system. As far as acid-base equilibrium
and pH regulation are concerned, the important substances in
the CSF are hydrogen ions, bicarbonate ions and carbon dioxide.
Of these three, only carbon dioxide, being lipid soluble, passes
readily between the blood and the cerebro-spinal fluid, so that the
cerebro-spinal fluid carbon dioxide tension rapidly follows that
of the plasma. This means that if the plasma P_{CO_2} increases for
any reason, the P_{CO_2} of the cerebro-spinal fluid also increases
equally, reaching equilibrium within a few minutes. Since the
CSF contains very little in the way of buffers apart from bicarbonate, the hydrogen ion concentration will rise about in
proportion to the rise in P_{CO_2}, so that doubling the P_{CO_2} will
lower the pH by 0.3 pH units. This is much more than the change
in pH of the plasma, since other buffers take up some of the
hydrogen ions released from the carbonic acid thus allowing the
formation of more free bicarbonate ions so that the bicarbonate
concentration also rises (reducing the change in the carbon dioxide: bicarbonate ratio – see Section 1.7). Similarly, a fall in
plasma P_{CO_2} will cause a rise in the pH of the cerebro-spinal fluid.
On the other hand, a change in the plasma hydrogen ion concentration will not have any direct effect on the pH of the cerebro-
spinal fluid, at least in the short term, since hydrogen ions do
not pass through the blood-brain barrier. If the pH of the cerebro-
spinal fluid does alter as a result of a long term maintained
alteration in the P_{CO_2} of the plasma, the cells of the choroid
plexus and other structures which secrete the cerebro-spinal fluid

alter the bicarbonate concentration in such a way as to restore the cerebro-spinal fluid to its normal pH. This could well be a result of processes similar to those which alter the pH and bicarbonate concentration of the fluid in the renal tubules, but the details are not known.

The significance of these changes in the pH of the CSF arises from the way in which the rate of respiration is controlled. As mentioned above the P_{CO_2} of the alveolar air depends on the rate at which CO_2 is being produced and on the alveolar ventilation. If, for example, the alveolar ventilation rate is doubled, provided the rate of production of carbon dioxide remains constant, the partial pressure of carbon dioxide will have halved when equilibrium is again reached.

Under normal conditions of metabolism at rest, the rate of alveolar ventilation is adjusted so that the P_{CO_2} in the arterial plasma remains constant. If even a very small change in P_{CO_2} occurs, an alteration of the ventilation rate so as to restore the P_{CO_2} follows. The change in alveolar ventilation occurs because nerve impulses arising from receptors which are sensitive to changes in chemical composition have reflex effects on the neurones which drive the respiratory movements. These chemically sensitive receptors are called chemoreceptors, and are functionally divided into two groups, the peripheral and the central chemoreceptors. (The peripheral receptors are located in the carotid and aertic bodies, and the central receptors somewhere in the medulla oblongata.)

The peripheral chemoreceptors increase their rate of firing in response to a rise in the P_{CO_2} or hydrogen ion concentration of the arterial plasma, and also respond if there is a considerable fall in the arterial oxygen partial pressure.

The central chemoreceptors appear to be sensitive only to the pH of the cerebro-spinal fluid which, as described above, is affected most rapidly by changes in arterial P_{CO_2}. The reflex responses driven by either of these sets of receptors increase the alveolar ventilation if the pH at either falls, but in terms of change of ventilation for unit change in pH, the system is much more sensitive to the central chemoreceptors.

3.3 *The Role of Respiration in pH Regulation*

If the P_{CO_2} of the plasma is raised, this will act on both the peripheral and central chemoreceptors so as to increase the alveolar ventilation. If the increased P_{CO_2} is maintained, as may occur in chronic respiratory disease, the drive to the respiratory centre diminishes because the pH of the cerebro-spinal fluid will gradually return towards normal as its bicarbonate concentration is raised following increased secretion of bicarbonate ions by the choroid plexus. In addition, the raised P_{CO_2} will increase the secretion of hydrogen ions into the renal tubules and hence increase the number of bicarbonate ions reabsorbed and so increase their concentration in the extracellular fluid. The pH of the extracellular fluid will therefore return towards normal (more slowly than the pH of the cerebro-spinal fluid does). Some stimulus to respiration is likely to remain, however, because a maintained rise in P_{CO_2} will usually be associated with a decreased alveolar ventilation so that the alveolar air will differ more from atmospheric air than usual, and not only is its P_{CO_2} raised, but its P_{O_2} is lowered. The arterial blood will therefore have a lower P_{O_2} and this will excite the peripheral chemoreceptors.

A situation which may occur in normal individuals is more or less the reverse of the above. This occurs when breathing air at a reduced atmospheric pressure at high altitude. Here the reduced partial pressure of oxygen in the inspired air, and hence in the arterial plasma, leads to stimulation of the peripheral chemoreceptors. Alveolar ventilation is increased and the P_{CO_2} of the alveolar air, and hence of the plasma, falls. This causes a rise in pH both in the plasma and in the cerebro-spinal fluid and this in turn tends to reduce the alveolar ventilation. However, the concentration of bicarbonate in the cerebro-spinal fluid will fall as a result of the activities of the choroid plexus and that of the plasma will fall as a result of decreased secretion of hydrogen ions by the renal tubules (and hence increased excretion of bicarbonate ions). A new equilibrium is reached with a raised alveolar ventilation rate, a (more or less) normal plasma and cerebro-spinal fluid pH, but with a reduced P_{CO_2} and bicarbonate concentration in both.

On return to normal atmospheric pressure, the lower P_{CO_2} is maintained, as any rise in it stimulates the respiration via both the peripheral and central chemoreceptors. The stimulus due to the low P_{O_2} has gone however, so the alveolar ventilation will be very slightly reduced and the P_{CO_2} will gradually rise again, since the rate of excretion of CO_2 will be very slightly less than its rate of production. As the P_{CO_2} rises, so will the secretion of hydrogen ions by the renal tubules and hence the reabsorption of bicarbonate ions, so that the concentration of bicarbonate in the extracellular fluid will also gradually rise. Equally, secretion of bicarbonate ions by the choroid plexus will increase so that the bicarbonate concentration in the CSF keeps pace with the rise in P_{CO_2}. This continues until the normal P_{CO_2} and bicarbonate concentrations have been regained.

In the preceding two examples, the changes in the plasma pH were produced as a result of a change in the P_{CO_2} following a change in the alveolar ventilation. The two conditions are therefore often referred to as 'respiratory acidosis' and 'respiratory alkalosis' respectively. If, on the other hand, a change in plasma pH is due to something other than a change in alveolar ventilation, it is referred to as a 'metabolic acidosis' or 'metabolic alkalosis' (even if not due to a change in metabolism).

If the pH of the plasma falls as a result of the addition of a certain amount of strong acid, this will lead to increased excitation of the peripheral chemoreceptors. This in turn will tend to increase the rate of alveolar ventilation and lower the plasma P_{CO_2}. However, lowering of the plasma P_{CO_2} leads to a lowering of the cerebro-spinal fluid P_{CO_2} and hence to an increase in its pH. This tends to cause a reduction in the alveolar ventilation and hence a rise in the P_{CO_2}. The peripheral and central chemoreceptors are tending to have opposite effects on the rate of alveolar ventilation, so the situation reached is a compromise, with the alveolar ventilation increased to the level where the effect of the central chemo-receptors due to the rise in CSF pH balances the effect of the peripheral chemoreceptors due to the fall in plasma pH. At equi-librium, the plasma will be partially restored towards its normal pH by the fall in P_{CO_2}. The fall in P_{CO_2} will reduce the rate of

secretion of bicarbonate ions into the CSF, so that the CSF bicarbonate will fall over the course of several hours. As the CSF bicarbonate falls, so will its pH (if the P_{CO_2} remains constant) and so the effect of the central chemoreceptors in tending to reduce the alveolar ventilation will be reduced. In fact, as this happens, the balance between the peripheral and central chemoreceptors will shift, so that there will be a progressive increase in alveolar ventilation (and hence a fall in P_{CO_2}) until a final equilibrium is reached (or would be reached in the absence of other mechanisms which restore the plasma pH) with the pH's of both plasma and CSF being slightly lower than normal, so that both peripheral and central chemoreceptors are tending to increase the alveolar ventilation to maintain the low P_{CO_2}. Since the fluids nevertheless still have a lower than normal pH, their bicarbonate concentrations must have been reduced in greater proportion than their P_{CO_2}, that of the CSF by reduced secretion of bicarbonate (and possibly by increased secretion of hydrogen ions) and that of the plasma (and extracellular fluid) as a result of having combined with some of the added hydrogen ions. Although the plasma pH may be very largely restored, the bicarbonate concentration and so the P_{CO_2} can only be restored by removing the hydrogen ions which were added. The hydrogen ions are excreted in the urine as a result of increased secretion by the cells of the distal convoluted tubules and collecting ducts. (It should also be noted that this description is only fully applicable to small or moderate amounts of acid or base being added. In severe disturbances of acid-base equilibrium, disturbances in, for example, the control of respiration may complicate the picture).

In 'metabolic alkalosis', as might be expected, the reverse changes will occur. A transient form of metabolic alkalosis occurs after every meal. Secretion of the acid gastric juice leads to bicarbonate ions entering the extracellular fluid, in the same way that secretion of hydrogen ions into the renal tubules leads to bicarbonate ions entering the extracellular fluid. 1 litre of gastric juice, which may be secreted following a meal, contains about 150 mEq of hydrogen ions. This secretion leads to the addition of 150 mEq of bicarbonate to the extracellular fluid and this

produces a rise in the bicarbonate concentration and hence in the pH. In fact, in man, the effect is quite small, since secretion of gastric juice is normally closely followed by the secretion of pancreatic juice. This has a much higher bicarbonate concentration than the extracellular fluid and so bicarbonate ions are disposed of into the gastro-intestinal tract before their production has finished and before any significant number have been excreted in the urine. Some animals, especially those which eat very large meals at long intervals have much larger alkaline tides than man. Following a meal, a small alligator, which eats about one quarter of its own weight every four or five days, may have an alkaline tide which raises its plasma pH to above 8, without very much effect on the urinary pH [12].

Some of the physiological buffering mechanisms are somewhat less effective for minimizing the effects of added alkali than they are for the effects of acid. A maintained rise in plasma pH will reduce the rate of firing of the peripheral chemoreceptors so that the rate of the alveolar ventilation will tend to fall. As in 'acidosis' the equilibrium reached will be set by the balance between the peripheral chemoreceptors responding to the rise of the plasma pH and the central chemoreceptors responding to the fall of CSF pH due to the rise in P_{CO_2}. Over the course of a few hours however, the CSF bicarbonate concentration will rise, allowing the equilibrium position to shift. However, as the alveolar ventilation is reduced, not only does the P_{CO_2} rise, but the P_{O_2} falls (as in 'respiratory acidosis'). The fall in P_{O_2} may eventually be sufficient to stimulate the peripheral chemoreceptors and will then tend to increase the ventilation. Thus the equilibrium finally reached (in the absence of the kidneys) would depend on the balance between raised pH and lowered P_{O_2} at the peripheral chemoreceptors in combination with the effect of the raised pH of the CSF. Because of this effect of low P_{O_2} the effectiveness of 'respiratory buffering' for alkali is likely to be somewhat less than it is for an equivalent amount of acid, particularly for large quantities. However, the end result of 'respiratory buffering' will be a return towards normal pH with a raised P_{CO_2} and an even greater rise (in proportion) in the bicarbonate concentration of both extracellular

fluid and CSF. The kidneys restore normal conditions by excreting urine which has a higher bicarbonate concentration (and pH) than plasma and disposing of the added hydroxyl ions in this form $(CO_2 + OH^- = HCO_3^-)$ as described in Section 3.4.

In summary, the addition of some acid to the extracellular fluid causes a small increase in ventilation, and hence a small fall in P_{CO_2}. The fall in P_{CO_2} increases over the course of several hours as the CSF bicarbonate concentration drops, allowing further increase in alveolar ventilation. Meanwhile, the kidneys start to secrete hydrogen ions into the urine, thus removing them from the body and allowing the plasma pH, bicarbonate concentration and P_{CO_2} to return to normal. This description, of course, relates to the artificial situation of a quantity of acid suddenly appearing in the body and also deals separately with the various stages of the amelioration of the effects of the acid and its ultimate disposal. In real life, acid does not appear suddenly in the body and the various processes for dealing with it take place concurrently with one another and with the production of the acid.

3.4 Hydrogen Ions and the Kidneys

The kidneys produce a large volume of glomerular filtrate which contains substances of low molecualr weight at concentrations more or less the same as those which they have in the plasma (see Section 2.7). In particular, the hydrogen ion concentration (or the pH) is almost the same. In the passage of the glomerular filtrate down the proximal tubules the volume falls to about 1/8 as a result of reabsorption. The pH remains roughly the same as that of the plasma, and hence the bicarbonate ion concentration is about the same as in the plasma. Thus the fluid reabsorbed must also have a pH and bicarbonate concentration similar to the plasma. The tubular walls are impermeable to bicarbonate ions, which therefore cannot be reabsorbed directly, but leave the tubules as CO_2 as a result of the active secretion of one hydrogen ion for each bicarbonate ion removed. (It has been suggested that there is a physical linkage between hydrogen ion

secretion and either potassium ion reabsorption or sodium ion reabsorption in the same sort of way as sodium extrusion and potassium reabsorption are linked in the 'sodium pump' in cell membranes. There is, however, little evidence either for or against the existence of such a linkage in the case of hydrogen ions. In either case, for the present discussion, it does not alter the overall effect).

The secretion of hydrogen ions tends to cause a shift in the equilibrium of the following reactions:

$$H^+ + HCO_3^- \rightleftharpoons H_2CO_3 \rightleftharpoons H_2O + CO_2 \qquad (3.1)$$

These reactions tend to go from left to right in the tubules (where the second reaction reaches equilibrium very quickly because of the presence of carbonic anhydrase in the brush border of the tubular cells). This tends to raise the P_{CO_2}, but the carbon dioxide diffuses through the tubular wall into the extracellular fluid, or into the tubular cells (where it makes these reactions tend to go back again from right to left). As the secretion of hydrogen ions probably more or less keeps pace with the reabsorption of water there would be very little actual change in the equilibrium within the tubules, even though the reaction is going continuously from left to right to keep constant the bicarbonate concentration of a shrinking volume of fluid.

Although the transport of many hydrogen ions takes place (against a small gradient) in the proximal tubules, so long as the bicarbonate concentration stays constant, it does not have very much effect on the acid-base equilibrium of the body as a whole, except in the sense that it does prevent the excretion of large numbers of bicarbonate ions in the urine. If a large proportion of the filtered bicarbonate ions were excreted, this would affect acid-base equilibrium, since the bicarbonate concentration of the urine would then exceed that of the plasma (since the volume of urine is very much less than the volume of glomerular filtrate) so the plasma bicarbonate would tend to fall. (The development of the mechanism for conserving bicarbonate must have been of very great importance in the evolution of reptiles from amphibia. Amphibia lose most of their metabolic carbon dioxide through the skin and have a low P_{CO_2} while reptiles excrete their carbon

dioxide through their lungs and so are similar to mammals).

The volume and pH of the fluid entering the distal tubules are little different from those of the fluid leaving the proximal tubules so little net movement of hydrogen ions or bicarbonate ions into or out of the fluid can have taken place in the loops of Henle.

In the distal tubules and collecting ducts, the main work of the kidneys in adjusting the final volume and composition of the urine takes place for hydrogen ions as for other substances. As far as acid-base equilibrium is concerned, the distal tubules and collecting ducts operate by secreting a number of hydrogen ions which can be adjusted over a wide range. The volume of fluid usually falls during its passage along the distal tubules and collecting ducts (unless the animal is producing its maximum possible urine flow). Since the tubular walls are impermeable to bicarbonate ions, the bicarbonate concentration will rise if no hydrogen ions are secreted. Since the P_{CO_2} remains constant, the pH would also rise. This would cause buffers in the fluid (mostly phosphate ions) to release hydrogen ions into solution. The hydrogen ions will combine with bicarbonate ions to produce carbon dioxide and water, thus reducing the quantity of bicarbonate somewhat (and reducing the change in pH).

If the distal tubules and collecting ducts do secrete some hydrogen ions into the tubular fluid, the final composition of the fluid will depend on the number of hydrogen ions secreted, the volume of the fluid and the quantity of buffers present. The only substances which are normally present in the fluid entering the distal tubules and which have any significant buffering action are bicarbonate ions and phosphate ions. The bicarbonate ions are, as described above, at roughly the same concentration as in the plasma, but the quantity of phosphate present depends on the amount of phosphate (or its metabolic precursors) absorbed from the diet. (Under normal circumstances, the quantity of phosphate in the body remains constant, so that the quantity excreted is the same as the quantity absorbed). The quantity of hydrogen ions that can be carried in the urine by the buffer systems is limited by their concentration and by the fact that the maximum gradient

between the extracellular fluid and the tubular fluid against which the tubular cells can transport hydrogen ions is about 1000:1. Since the pH of the extracellular fluid is normally 7.4, the lowest pH that the urine can reach is about 4.4. Whatever the final pH, the net number of hydrogen ions lost to the body, both free and in combination with phosphate and bicarbonate and other buffers can be determined by measuring (e.g. by titration) how many hydrogen ions have to be removed (or added for an alkaline urine) to bring the pH back to that of the extracellular fluid. In order to get a reliable estimate of the number of hydrogen ions which have combined with bicarbonate ions, the titration must be carried out at the P_{CO_2} of the extracellular fluid. The quantity determined in this way is often referred to as the 'titratable acid' of the urine (but see below).

In an acid urine, since the tubular wall is permeable to carbon dioxide, the bicarbonate concentration will be reduced in the same proportion that the hydrogen ion concentration is raised, because from the equilibrium of the reactions of equation (3.1).

$$[HCO_3^-] = \frac{K[CO_2]}{[H^+]} \quad \text{(see also Section 1.7)}$$

However, the right hand reaction of equation (3.1) takes some time to reach equilibrium in the absence of a catalyst. There is no carbonic anhydrase in the luminal walls of the distal tubular cells (unlike those of the proximal tubules) and the ureters and bladder are impermeable to carbon dioxide. Equilibrium will not have been reached by the time the urine leaves the collecting ducts so that the P_{CO_2} and bicarbonate concentration of an acid urine in the bladder will be somewhat higher than their equilibrium values. (Also, especially when excreting a concentrated urine, the P_{CO_2} in the renal medulla is somewhat higher than in the extracellular fluid as a whole – see Section 2.9). Even so, in an acid urine, the bicarbonate concentration will be low and so will the buffering capacity of the bicarbonate (although each bicarbonate ion which has been removed as CO_2 has removed, and so in a sense has buffered a hydrogen ion). The buffering capacity of the phosphate ions in the urine would be adequate

to maintain acid-base equilibrium of a person on a normal mixed Western diet, but would provide no reserve 'acid-excreting capacity'. Reserve capacity is provided by the ability of the cells of the distal tubules and collecting ducts to synthesize ammonia, which diffuses into the tubular fluid where it forms ammonium ions by combining with hydrogen ions. In an acid urine, the pH is very far from the pK of the dissociation of ammonium ions (see Section 2.10), so the ammonia is a very poor buffer in the usual sense. However, very nearly every ammonia molecule which enters the tubular fluid combines with a hydrogen ion and removes it from solution, whatever the urinary pH within the physiological range. Thus, for each ammonia molecule produced by the kidneys and excreted in the urine, a hydrogen ion can be removed from the body in a form in which it affects the acid-base equilibrium of the body but has virtually no effect on the pH of the urine. This means that the synthesis of ammonia allows more hydrogen ions to be removed at a given hydrogen ion concentration gradient between the extracellular fluid and the tubular fluid. This would reduce the energy required to transport the hydrogen ions into the tubules for a certain number of hydrogen ions excreted and increase the number of hydrogen ions that can be transported against the maximum gradient which the tubular cells can generate (i.e. when the pH of the urine is about 4.4).

The presence of ammonia thus increases the number of hydrogen ions which can be excreted in the urine. It also means that the net excretion of hydrogen ions cannot be estimated simply by titrating the urine back to a pH of 7.4, since nearly all the hydrogen ions combined with ammonia at the pH of the urine will remain combined with ammonia at a pH of 7.4; for each 99 999 hydrogen ions combined with ammonia at a pH of 4.4 only 999 or just under 1% will have dissociated at a pH of 7.4, and the proportion will be even smaller if the initial pH is higher. However, the total excretion can readily be determined. Titration is used to determine the number of excreted hydrogen ions free and in combination with buffers other than ammonia, while the number in combination with ammonia is very nearly the same as the total number of ammonia molecules (as NH_3 and NH_4^+)

present, which can be determined separately.

3.5 *Abnormal Metabolism*

Under unusual conditions of metabolism, there may be short or long term disturbances of acid-base equilibrium. The most familiar of these is during severe muscular exercise. The metabolism of glucose provides the energy for muscles, and the complete metabolism of glucose to carbon dioxide and water is, as described above, a neutral reaction as far as the acid-base equilibrium of the body is concerned. However, this complete metabolism needs oxygen and, in the absence of sufficient oxygen, energy is provided by the metabolic breakdown of glucose to lactic acid. This provides much less energy per molecule of glucose, so large amounts of lactic acid may be formed and enter the extracellular fluid. Lactic acid is a fairly strong acid (with a pK of about 3.8) so nearly all of it will be dissociated at a pH of 7.4 and the resulting hydrogen ions will have to be removed from solution. The body's capacity for exercise of this severity is limited before sufficient lactic acid has been produced to seriously overload the short-term buffering mechanisms by, among other things, the development of pain in the active muscles. On stopping the severe exercise, when sufficient oxygen is again available, lactic acid is rapidly resynthesized to glucose or glycogen and the energy to do this is provided by metabolizing some of the lactic acid to carbon dioxide and water. Thus the hydrogen ions released by the lactic acid (or rather an equivalent number of hydrogen ions) are taken out of solution in combination with the lactate ions from which they had earlier dissociated. This raises the pH, and the hydrogen ions taken up by the buffers are released again. In this way, the acid-base equilibrium is restored metabolically after only a relatively short-term and transient disturbance.

In some metabolic disorders there may be long-term factors affecting acid-base balance. This is particularly marked where an adequate supply of glucose is not available as a source of metabolic energy (in particular for the central nervous system), such as occurs

in diabetes mellitus or total starvation. In these circumstances, fat is used as a major source of energy and, although the complete oxidative metabolism of fat gives rise to carbon dioxide and water, in the absence of glucose, among the end-products of fat metabolism are β hydroxy-butyric acid and aceto-acetic acid, the so-called keto acids. These are both quite strong acids and therefore dissociate almost completely at the pH of the tissue fluids, giving rise to many hydrogen ions which, in order to maintain acid-base equilibrium, must be removed temporarily by the buffering systems and finally by the kidneys. Some of the keto acid anions are metabolized to carbon dioxide and water, which (as with the metabolism of lactic acid) removes an equivalent number of hydrogen ions. Some are converted from the form of the undissociated acid into acetone:

$$CH_3-CO-CH_2-COOH \longrightarrow CH_3-CO-CH_3 + CO_2$$

so again effectively removing a hydrogen ion for each molecule of acetone formed. However, especially in diabetes mellitus, the acids are produced more rapidly than they can be removed by these metabolic activities. They therefore tend to accumulate as β hydroxy-butyrate and acetoacetate ions in the extracellular fluid and plasma. Since the ions are of low molecular weight, they will pass into the tubular fluid in the glomeruli of the kidneys and will hence be excreted in the urine. The rate of loss will increase with the concentration in the plasma until equilibrium is reached, with the rate of loss being equal to the rate of production. At the minimum possible urinary pH (about 4.4), about half the β hydroxy-butyrate and the majority of the aceto-acetate will still be ionized since their pKs are about 4.4 and 3.6 respectively. This means that the majority of the hydrogen ions from the original acids have to be excreted either free or in combination with other buffers and ammonium ions — see Section 3.4. In addition the keto acid anions will need to be balanced by an equivalent number of cations. In starvation, the rate of production of keto-acids is not so great that the kidneys cannot excrete their hydrogen ions in this way, but in severe diabetes the kidneys can no longer keep pace, and the free hydrogen ion content of the

body rises, together with the number of hydrogen ions taken up by the buffers. An equilibrium no longer exists, so the (free) hydrogen ion concentration rises, eventually to a level which is not compatible with life.

Another problem resulting from the metabolic abnormalities which occur in diabetes arises from the increased quantities of solutes in the urine. The raised plasma glucose concentration means that a greater quantity of glucose than normal enters the renal tubules in the glomerular filtrate and this quantity will be greater than the transport maximum for glucose. If the plasma glucose concentration remained at 17 mmol l^{-1} (3 g l^{-1}) over the course of 24 hours — it might average about this in a relatively mild diabetes — then about 3 mol of glucose would enter the 180 l of glomerular filtrate formed. The T_m for glucose is about 300 mg min^{-1} (see Fig. 4 in Section 2.6) or about 1.7 mmol min^{-1}, which is about 2.4 mol per day. Thus about 0.6 mol of glucose will not be reabsorbed from the renal tubules and so will be excreted in the urine. Since glucose is not ionized in solution this represents an extra 600 mmol of solute particles in the urine. In addition to this there is the quantity of any keto acid anions and the associated cations which may appear in the urine.

If the body is to remain in equilibrium, these solutes plus the 'normal' solutes produced from the diet (i.e. salts, urea etc.) must be excreted in the urine. This greatly increases the solute load, which reduces the maximum concentration of the urine and considerably increases its minimum volume (see Section 2.9). A considerably increased water intake is therefore necessary to make up for the increased urinary output, otherwise the body's content of water will fall. (Indeed, the term diabetes is derived from Greek words which describe the greatly increased through-put of fluids. Even before the days of chemical analysis of the urine, two forms of diabetes could be distringuished. In diabetes mellitus, the increase in urine volume is due to the large amount of glucose in the urine, so that the urine tastes sweet (mellitus from the Latin for honey). In diabetes insipidus, the large volume of urine is a result of the kidneys not being able to reabsorb water from the distal convoluted tubules and collecting ducts, so that

the urine is very dilute and tastes insipid.)

Once a diabetic (i.e. a sufferer from diabetes mellitus) becomes comatose, primarily as a result of the falling pH of the body fluids, his water intake ceases, so he will no longer be taking sufficient fluid to replace the water lost in the urine. The volume of the body fluids will fall which will lead to a fall in the systemic arterial pressure and hence to a fall in the glomerular filtration rate. This will, among other things, impair the kidneys' ability to excrete hydrogen ions in the urine, so that the pH of the body fluids will fall even faster. Thus, if someone has diabetes sufficiently severe to make him comatose, his metabolism must quickly be restored to normal (by insulin) if he is to survive.

3.5 *Secondary Effects of and Recovery from Severe Metabolic Acidosis*

Changes in the metabolism may give rise to marked changes in the acid-base equilibrium, most commonly in an acid direction. This may lead to an equilibrium being reached with the hydrogen ion concentration of the extracellular fluid higher than normal, or equilibrium may not be reached, and the hydrogen ion concentration continues to rise until death occurs, as in untreated severe diabetes. As the hydrogen ion concentration gradually rises, the extracellular buffer ratios and respiration will change, as has already been described. In addition, the hydrogen ion concentration inside the cells will also rise. The great majority of the hydrogen ions entering the cells will combine with protein or other buffers — mostly phosphate ions and organic ions. In order to maintain the charge on the inside of the cell, for each hydrogen ion that enters the cell, either another positively charged ion must leave the cell, or a negatively charged ion must enter. In fact, some of each happens (see Section 1.10) and certainly some potassium ions leave the cells. This lowers the potassium concentration in the cells and tends to raise the potassium concentration in the extra-cellular fluid. Potassium ions also diffuse in greater numbers from the cells of the renal tubules into the

tubular fluid so that much potassium is lost in the urine, and there may, in fact, be little or no rise in the extracellular fluid potassium concentration. Even so, the intracellular-extracellular concentration ratio for potassium will fall, and so the membrane potential of the cells will also fall. The end result is that the intracellular and extracellular hydrogen ion concentration rises and the intracellular potassium concentration falls, and some or all of the potassium which is lost from the cells is excreted in the urine so that the total body content of potassium will also fall.

When in diabetes normal metabolism is restored by insulin, the production of keto acids ceases, and those still present in the body will be metabolized to carbon dioxide and water. The intracellular and extracellular pH is still low initially, so that the kidneys continue to excrete a highly acid urine containing a high concentration of ammonium salts, so that hydrogen ions are now being removed from the body more rapidly than they are being produced. The bicarbonate ions manufactured by the kidneys (as a result of the excretion of hydrogen ions) enter the plasma and the majority very rapidly combine with free hydrogen ions. This will lead to the release of further hydrogen ions by the dissociation of other buffers. The carbonic acid so produced will mostly be excreted via the lungs, as carbon dioxide. In this way a restoration of the normal pH and buffer system ratios (and bicarbonate concentration) occurs in the extracellular fluid. This leads to a net movement of hydrogen ions into the extracellular fluid from the cells, since the ions will now be diffusing in more slowly, although they are still being pumped out at the same rate. Most of these hydrogen ions have been in combination with buffers inside the cells, so that the intracellular buffer systems also start to return to their normal ratios. However, for each hydrogen ion that leaves the cell, either a negative ion must leave or a positive ion must enter and, in fact, in a manner similar to what happened when the intracellular pH was falling, some of the each will occur.

The extracellular fluid contains a relatively low concentration of potassium ions. Since many of the potassium ions which passed

from the cells into the extracellular fluid as the pH was falling have been excreted in the urine, there will not be sufficient potassium ions in the extracellular fluid to enable the intracellular potassium concentration to be restored to normal. However, the cells will take up some of those that are in the extracellular fluid, leading to a fall in the potassium concentration here (and a proportionally very much smaller rise in the intracellular potassium concentration), which will increase the intracellular-extracellular potassium concentration ratio to above its normal value. This means that the membrane potential will become higher than normal which will make the outward transport of hydrogen ions more difficult (as well as encouraging their inward diffusion) and will also affect the distribution of other ions. Thus even after the extracellular pH has been restored to normal, the pH inside the cells will still be low, including the cells of the renal tubules. The tubule cells will therefore continue to synthesize ammonia and to secrete hydrogen ions into the tubules. (In the absence of sufficient sodium ions in the urine to balance the non-reabsorbable anions, the excretion of hydrogen ions will also be encouraged by the tubular cells endeavouring to reabsorb as many potassium ions as possible from the urine). Thus the bicarbonate concentration and the pH of the extracellular fluid will continue to rise, to above their normal levels. The only way by which the normal state of affairs can be restored is by supplying the body with sufficient potassium to enable the cells to restore their potassium concentration to normal. This will allow the excess intracellular hydrogen ions back into the extracellular fluid, where they can be removed by combining with the bicarbonate ions produced by the renal tubules as they continue to excrete hydrogen ions into the urine.

4. Salt and Water Balance

4.1 *Introduction*

The extracellular fluid provides the environment in which most of the cells of the body live, and the continuance of their normal activities is dependent upon the maintenance of a relatively constant composition for their environment. One of the important factors which must be controlled is the total osmotic concentration of the extracellular fluid since the total osmotic concentration inside the cells depends on this. Quantitatively very much the most abundant solutes of the extracellular fluid (in terms of moles or equivalents per litre) are sodium salts — mostly sodium chloride and sodium bicarbonate. Because sodium salts make up such a high proportion of the solute particles, the osmotic concentration of the extracellular fluid depends very largely upon the total concentration of sodium ions (+ of course, their associated anions) so that if the sodium concentration is adequately controlled then the osmotic pressure will be adequately controlled also.

Although the activities of the cells are very much affected by the composition and osmotic concentration of the extracellular fluid, the actual volume of the fluid is less important, at least as far as an individual cell is concerned. However, large changes in the volume of the extracellular fluid will have mechanical effects on the tissues (as illustrated by the changes in the skin and sub-cutaneous tissues detectable as oedema, or, at the other extreme, the stiffness and inelasticity of these tissues when the volume of extracellular fluid is much reduced as in 'dehydration'). In addition the plasma is a part of the extracellular fluid, and changes in the total volume of the extracellular fluid are normally associated with parallel changes in the volume of the plasma. Any marked change in plasma volume will affect the operation of the cardio-vascular system and so have effects on the body as a whole. Thus

as far as the individual cells are concerned, small fluctuations in the volume of the extracellular fluid will be of less significance than small fluctuations in its osmotic concentration, although both volume and osmotic pressure must be controlled.

In any solution the osmotic concentration depends on the concentration of solute — i.e. the quantity per unit volume of solution. Thus, for a given volume of solvent, the osmotic concentration is directly proportional to the quantity of solute present, while, for a given quantity of solute, the osmotic concentration is inversely proportional to the volume of solvent. However, if the quantities of both solvent and solute change in proportion, the osmotic concentration remains constant. The same argument applies to the extracellular fluid in the body. If the quantities of sodium salts and water in the extracellular fluid change in the right proportion to each other, then the osmotic concentration of the extracellular fluid will remain constant. This is equivalent to a net gain or loss of fluid isotonic to the extracellular fluid. There are many possible combinations of water gain or loss and sodium salt gain or loss, but they will all give rise to changes in the osmotic concentration and/or the volume of the extracellular fluid. The kidneys are involved in the mechanisms for preventing or minimizing such changes, or, if they have occurred, in assisting to restore the extracellular fluid to its normal volume and osmotic concentration. They are able to do this because the final osmotic concentration and the sodium salt content of the urine can be altered relatively independently of each other.

In order to maintain salt and water balance, it is necessary to ensure that over a period the quantities leaving the body are the same as the quantities entering. (Obviously, as food and drink are not taken continuously, there are bound to be fluctuations in the balance in the short term.) Although salts and water are lost from the body by a number of different routes, the quantities lost by routes other than the kidney depend mainly upon environmental factors, and so are much less easily regulated than the quantities lost in the urine. Changes in the overall sodium salt or water content of the body will, as described above, give rise to

alterations of the osmotic concentration and/or the volume of the extracellular fluid. This means that the maintenance of the salt and water balance of the body is equivalent to maintenance of the osmotic concentration and volume of the extracellular fluid. The mechanisms which the body has for controlling the operations of kidneys so as to help to maintain salt and water balance in fact operate (as described below) by monitoring the osmotic concentration and the volume of the extracellular fluid, and these mechanisms are relatively independent of each other. It is therefore convenient, at least initially, to describe these mechanisms separately.

4.2 *Regulation of Osmotic Concentration*

The kidneys start their operations by the formation of large volumes of glomerular filtrate which, as mentioned previously (Section 2.7) has virtually the same composition, and hence the same osmotic concentration, as the extracellular fluid in most tissues of the body. A very large proportion of this fluid is re-absorbed, but if the urine finally produced has an osmotic concentration different from that of the glomerular filtrate, it means that the osmotic concentration of the fluid reabsorbed must also differ from that of the glomerular filtrate (but by a much smaller amount and in the opposite direction). Thus, if the urine has a higher osmotic concentration, then the reabsorbed fluid must have a lower osmotic concentration than the glomerular filtrate, and hence a lower osmotic concentration than the extracellular fluid. This will tend to cause the osmotic concentration of the extracellular fluid to fall.

To take a specific example, suppose that in a day a man secretes 500 ml of urine with an osmotic concentration of 1200 mmol l^{-1}. (The highly concentrated urine indicates that much antidiuretic hormone is present in the plasma, which in turn suggests that the osmotic concentration of the extracellular fluid is high, see below). This urine is made up of 500 ml of water which contains 600 mmol of solute particles. The glomerular fil-

trate formed in a day has a volume of 180 l and an osmotic concentration (assuming that it remains constant throughout the day) of 300 mmol l^{-1}. Hence it would contain a total of 54 000 mmol of solutes. Since only 500 ml of water and 600 mmol of solutes remain in the urinary tract, 179.5 litres of water and 53 400 mmol of solutes would have been reabsorbed. This fluid would have an osmotic concentration of 53 400/179.5, which is 297.5 mmol l^{-1}. This shows that the fluid reabsorbed does have a lower osmotic concentration than the extracellular fluid, although its osmotic concentration differs from it only very slightly, while that of the urine differs very much more, because of its much smaller volume. The effect this would have on the body as a whole is very difficult to appreciate from these figures, and is much easier to visualize by looking at them in a different way.

To see what effect this could have on the osmotic concentration of the body fluids (assuming the impossible situation that no water or solutes were gained or lost by any other route during the 24 hours), the 500 ml of water and 600 mmol of solutes which together make up the urine can be dealt with separately. If the man is considered to start with a total of 50 litres of body fluid (both extracellular and intracellular) with an osmotic concentration of 300 mmol l^{-1}, i.e. a total of 15 000 mmol, then he will finish up with 49.5 l containing 14 400 mmol of solutes. This will have an osmotic concentration of 14 400/49.5 which is 291 mmol l^{-1}. Thus the secretion of 500 ml of urine with an osmotic concentration of 1200 mmol l^{-1} or 4 times the concentration of the extracellular fluid, will, under these highly simplified and artificial conditions, reduce the osmotic concentration of the body fluids by about 9 mmol l^{-1}, or about 3%, over the course of 24 hours.

The effect of secreting such a urine can also be appreciated by thinking of the urine as being formed from a volume of fluid containing the same quantity of solutes as the urine secreted, but with the same osmotic concentration as the extracellular fluid. (This is in effect what happens as the urine passes down the collecting ducts from the distal convoluted tubules to the pelvis of the ureter). Taking this particular example, 600 mmol

of solutes are contained in 2 l of extracellular fluid, so that to produce 500 ml of urine, 1500 ml of water (without any solutes) must have been reabsorbed as the fluid passed down the collecting ducts. This water is available to reduce the osmotic concentration of the body fluids, as described above. However, it is important to remember that this water has not really been 'gained' by the body, even though the osmotic concentration of the body fluids has been reduced. In fact 500 ml of water has been lost from the body to carry the 'extra' solutes to make this 1500 ml available.

Precisely parallel changes, but in the opposite sense, will occur in the body when a urine with a lower osmotic concentration than the extracellular fluid is secreted. Effects of approximately the same magnitude as those described above would be produced if the man secreted 3.5 l of urine with an osmotic concentration of 171 mmol l^{-1} in 24 hours. This represents 3.5 l of water containing 600 mmol of solutes, so that the same quantity of solutes is contained in 1.5 l more instead of 1.5 l less than the volume of extracellular fluid which contains the same quantity of solutes.

From the above it can be seen that the kidneys, by secreting a urine with an osmotic concentration different from that of the extracellular fluid are potentially able to produce quite considerable changes in its osmotic concentration over a period. The changes in osmotic concentration of the urine are, as mentioned above (Sections 2.9, 2.12) a result of the action of antidiuretic hormone on the kidneys — the greater the amount of antidiuretic hormone which is circulating in the blood, the higher the concentration of the urine (within the limits which the kidneys can reach with the quantity of solutes present in the urine at the time). Large concentrations of antidiuretic hormone will tend to lead to a reduction of the osmotic concentration of the body fluids and vice versa. This suggests that a raised osmotic concentration in the body fluids should lead to increased release of antidiuretic hormone, and this is indeed so. The cells of the supra-optic nuclei of the hypothalamus are sensitive (perhaps indirectly) to changes in osmotic concentration and, in response to a rise in osmotic concentration, increase the rate at which they discharge nerve impulses [17]. This increase in firing rate leads to an increase in

the rate of release of antidiuretic hormone from the terminals of these cells which lie in the posterior lobe of the pituitary gland. This in turn leads to reabsorption from the renal tubules of fluid which has a lower osmotic concentration than the extracellular fluid and hence tends to lower the osmotic concentration of the body fluids. Conversely, a fall in the osmotic concentration reduces the rate of discharge of these neurones, and hence reduces the rate of secretion of antidiuretic hormone, leading to the secretion of a urine of low osmotic concentration and hence to an increase in the osmotic concentration of the body fluids. Thus changes in osmotic concentration lead indirectly to changes in the operation of the kidneys which tend to restore the osmotic concentration to normal.

As well as leading to changes in the quantity of circulating antidiuretic hormone, the action on the hypothalamus of an altered osmotic concentration also leads to alteration in the fluid intake by altering the 'appetite' for fluids. (Although, when water is freely available, many animals regulate their fluid intake in anticipation of likely changes in the osmotic concentration of their extracellular fluid, rather than in respect to changes which have already taken place [18].) For instance a rise in the osmotic concentration of the body fluids gives rise to a sensation of thirst, which, if suitable fluid is available, can be expected to lead to an increased fluid intake, and if the fluid has a lower osmotic concentration (in terms of non-metabolized solutes), its absorption from the gastro-intestinal tract will tend to reduce the osmotic concentration of the body fluids. Water intake may be very accurately controlled by thirst; some animals, e.g. camels and donkeys, drink in a very short time following a period of water deprivation, a quantity of water which when it has been absorbed, will exactly restore the body fluids to their normal concentration [39]. The regulation of fluid intake by the hypothalamus makes it possible to regulate the osmotic concentration of the body fluids reasonably well, even without the ability to alter the con- centration of the urine, which will occur for example, when no antidiuretic hormone is produced, as in diabetes insipidus.

The hypothalamus appears to be sensitive to stimuli other than

a change in the osmotic concentration of the plasma, since other factors are able to alter the rate of secretion of antidiuretic hormone and the thirst, although the effects of changes in osmotic concentration are usually much larger, particularly in the long term. A change which causes an increased secretion of antidiuretic hormone is a reduction in the volume of the extracellular fluid, particularly the plasma. This gives rise to the sensation of thirst and the reduction in the rate of urine secretion which occurs particularly after haemorrhage, and which will help to restore the volume of the extracellular fluid, or at least reduce its rate of diminution, at the expense of slightly reducing its osmotic concentration. The reverse changes occur with an increase in the extracellular fluid volume, so that the excess fluid is removed somewhat more rapidly than the solutes dissolved in it, which means that the volume is reduced at the expense of a small rise in osmotic concentration. Such changes in extracellular fluid volume produce parallel alterations in the rate of secretion of aldosterone, which is dealt with more fully in the next Section.

The relatively much greater sensitivity to osmotic concentration than to extracellular fluid volume is illustrated by the difference in the responses of a normal man between drinking a large volume of water and a large volume of sodium chloride solution isotonic with the extracellular fluid. Absorbing 1 litre of water from the gut would produce about a 2% fall in osmotic concentration and a 2% rise in extracellular fluid volume (since the water will be distributed amongst all the body fluid, both intracellular and extracellular). This produces a great reduction in the rate of antidiuretic hormone secretion and a considerable rise in the rate of urine flow so that most of the water is excreted in the urine within 2 − 3 hours. Absorbing a litre of normal saline will produce no change in osmotic concentration and it will all remain in the extracellular fluid, so will produce about a 5% rise in extracellular fluid volume. However, since there is usually only a small change in the rate of secretion of urine, it can have had little effect on the rate of antidiuretic hormone secretion. There is a gradual rise in the quantity of sodium salts in the urine, so that it usually takes at least 12 hours and often more to excrete all the water and

sodium chloride which has been absorbed.

Other factors which frequently increase the rate of secretion of antidiuretic hormone are exercise, fright and sleep. For the former two, this may be thought of as retaining water in advance in case it is needed for sweat to cool the exercising body, while in sleep it reduces the likelihood of needing to wake up to urinate.

By a combination of alterations of the final osmotic concentration of the urine and of the amount of fluid drunk, the osmotic concentration of the body fluids is controlled within narrow limits under a wide range of external environmental conditions. Both the 'internal' mechanism (i.e. via antidiuretic hormone) and the 'external' mechanism (i.e. alterations of fluid intake) which are mediated via the hypothalamus are quite powerful and rapidly acting and either can maintain a constant osmotic concentration on its own, but either on its own is less effective, especially under adverse external conditions, than the two acting together (see also Sections 4.5 and 4.6).

4.3 *Regulation of Extracellular Fluid Volume*

Because the osmotic concentration of the body fluids is normally closely controlled, the total volume of the extracellular fluid depends almost entirely upon the total quantity of sodium ions which it contains. This means that alteration of the extracellular fluid volume may be achieved by altering the total quantity of sodium salts in the extracellular fluid. (Since the great majority of the sodium ions in the body are in the extracellular fluid this is almost equivalent to altering the total quantity of sodium salts in the body as a whole). Under normal circumstances, the great majority of the sodium salts present in the diet are absorbed from the gut, and the kidneys form the only route by which large quantities leave the body, although small amounts of sodium salts also leave in the sweat and the faeces. In a hot environment, where large amounts of sweat are secreted in the process of keeping the body temperature down, the amount of sodium salts lost in the sweat may indeed be quite large and of great significance to the

salt balance of the body (see Section 4.4).

In order to maintain constant the sodium ion content of the body and hence the volume of the extracellular fluid, it is only necessary to ensure that the quantity of sodium ions excreted is the same as the quantity absorbed (or rather, the quantity absorbed, less the quantity leaving the body by routes other than the kidneys). There appears to be no direct way of regulating the quantity absorbed, so that the only way of determining the quantity which has to be excreted is by detecting the quantity that has already been absorbed. If, over a period, more sodium ions have been absorbed than have been excreted, the sodium content of the body will rise, and so will the volume of the extracellular fluid (provided the osmotic concentration remains constant). This rise in the volume of the extracellular fluid indicates the need to excrete more sodium ions, so that an increase in volume should lead to an increase in the rate at which sodium ions are excreted. Similarly, a decrease in the volume of the extracellular fluid should lead to a reduction in the sodium ion excretion.

In man, the major factor which alters the rate of sodium ion excretion is an alteration in the concentration of aldosterone (and to a much smaller extent that of some other steroid hormones) in the plasma. As described above (Section 2.12), an increase in the aldosterone level causes an increase in the quantity of sodium ions which are reabsorbed in the distal convoluted tubules and collecting ducts, so reducing the quantity of sodium ions which appear in the urine. (Aldosterone also increases to a relatively small extent the reabsorption of sodium ions by the ascending limbs of the loops of Henle, thus increasing the maximum concentration of urine which the kidneys can produce). In some animals, e.g. the dog, an increase in the rate of sodium ion excretion is associated with an increase in the glomerular filtration rate. This will increase the rate at which sodium ions enter the renal tubules, so that unless the rate of reabsorption of sodium ions from the tubules increases in parallel (which in these circumstances it does not), the number of sodium ions remaining in the tubular fluid and being excreted will also increase. Following a

large protein meal, however, the dog (and other carnivores) may also have a considerable increase in glomerular filtration rate. This leads to an increase in the rate of urea excretion, but under these circumstances, the rate of sodium ion reabsorption in the proximal tubules appears to increase more or less in parallel with the rise in glomerular filtration rate, so that there is little increase in the rate of sodium excretion. In man and many other non-carnivores, the glomerular filtration rate is very much less variable than in the dog. However, there is some evidence that sodium ion excretion may be altered in some species, e.g. the rat, and perhaps also in man, by reducing the glomerular filtration rate in some ('sodium-conserving') nephrons and increasing it in other ('sodium-losing') nephrons without much alteration in the total glomerular filtration rate [24]. It is still necessary to adjust the rate of aldosterone secretion or the glomerular filtration rate according to the volume of the extracellular fluid to enable either of these two mechanisms to operate successfully. In the case of aldosterone, since a rise in its concentration leads to an increased reabsorption, and hence a reduced excretion of sodium ions, a rise in the extracellular fluid volume should lead to a reduction in the aldosterone secretion and vice versa. In those species which alter their glomerular filtration rate, a rise in the extracellular fluid volume should lead to a rise in the glomerular filtration rate (without a parallel rise in sodium reabsorption). Aldosterone secretion is also directly affected by the composition of the plasma of the blood passing through the adrenal gland. A reduced concentration of sodium ions or a raised concentration of potassium ions leads to an increase in the rate of secretion [15].

As mentioned above, a change in the volume of the extracellular fluid will normally be associated with a change in the same direction in the volume of the plasma and hence in the total blood volume. It appears that alterations in the glomerular filtration rate and in the rate of aldosterone secretion occur in response to effects produced by changes in the total blood volume. Although some mechanisms involved seem to be reasonably well established, and are described below, the picture is almost certainly very far from complete.

The cardiovascular system is a closed system, and for these purposes can be considered to consist of the arteries and the veins, connected by a series of capillary systems which have a relatively constant volume. The arterial system consists of relatively stiff but elastic vessels containing blood at high pressure. An increase in the volume of blood contained in these vessels will therefore stretch their walls and as a result increase the pressure within them (and vice versa for a fall in volume). The venous system on the other hand consists of vessels with relatively thin pliable walls containing blood at a low pressure. An increase in the volume of blood in the veins will distend them, but not lead to any great increase in pressure, and a fall in volume will lead to less distension but again little change in pressure. Thus a change in the volume of blood in the circulatory system as a whole would be expected to affect both the venous and the arterial sides of the circulation — the most prominent effect on the venous side being an alteration in distension and on the arterial side being an alteration in pressure. The precise balance between the changes in the two parts of the circulatory system is not just a result of purely physical processes, since an alteration in volume (or pressure) in either part also affects the various reflex mechanisms which control the circulatory system. As far as aldosterone is concerned, there is evidence that distension of the right atrium or the veins of the head and neck leads to a decreased secretion and hence to an increased excretion of sodium ions in the urine. The mechanism by which the aldosterone secretion is altered is not known. Changes in the arterial pressure are detected in the kidneys themselves. The juxta-glomerular apparatus appears to be able to so regulate the diameter of the afferent arteriole leading to the corresponding glomerulus that the pressure in the glomerular capillaries remains relatively constant despite considerable changes in the arterial pressure (Section 2.7). They must therefore be sensitive to changes in arterial pressure, and, in response to a fall in arterial pressure, they release an enzyme called renin into the blood. Renin acts on certain proteins in the plasma to split off a substance known as angiotensin I which is in turn converted by another enzyme in the plasma into angiotensin II. Angiotensin II

causes the adrenal glands to release aldosterone into the plasma.
Thus a fall in blood volume, leading to a fall in arterial pressure,
causes the juxta-glomerular apparatus to increase the rate of
release of renin, which in turn leads to an increase in the rate of
release of aldosterone. In this way, a fall in extracellular fluid
volume leads eventually to an increase in the reabsorption of
sodium ions from the renal tubules, and hence to a reduction in
the excretion of sodium ions.

If the juxta-glomerular apparatus did not fully 'autoregulate'
the blood pressure in the glomerular capillaries in response to a
rise in arterial pressure, this would give rise to an increase in the
glomerular filtration rate (see Section 2.7). This does not appear
to happen even in the dog, where a rise in arterial pressure on its
own produces no change in the glomerular filtration rate, although
an increase in sodium excretion may be associated with a very
large increase in the filtration rate. The mechanism by which
autoregulation takes place is not yet known, but there is some
evidence which suggests that the juxta-glomerular apparatus may
be able to alter the calibre of the afferent arteriole in response
to changes in sodium ion concentration in the tubular fluid in
the distal convoluted tubule where it comes into contact with
the juxta-glomerular apparatus [40]. A rise in the sodium concentration here would be expected to occur following an increase
in the glomerular filtration rate in the nephron, since the
relatively constant rate of reabsorption of sodium ions in the
preceding parts of the nephron will have removed a smaller proportion of the increased number of sodium ions entering the
tubule. In this way it would be possible for the glomerular
filtration rate to be regulated by adjusting the afferent arteriole
in response to changes in the sodium concentration of the tubular
fluid passing the juxta-glomerular apparatus. If the filtration rate
in the nephron increased, this would increase the sodium concentration in the distal convoluted tubule which would make the
afferent arteriole constrict. This would increase its resistance to
flow and so reduce the flow of blood into and the pressure within the glomerular capillaries and thus reduce the glomerular
filtration rate again. If this is indeed how the juxta-glomerular

apparatus operates, the increase in filtration rate associated with an increase in sodium excretion as occurs in the dog, cannot be a direct result of an increase in arterial pressure. It must depend on some other factor which alters the relationship which the juxta-glomerular apparatus maintains between afferent arteriole diameter and distal convoluted tubule sodium ion concentration.

Changes in the volume of blood in the heart and veins of the head, and changes of arterial pressure may occur even in the absence of an overall change in the volume of the blood or extracellular fluid. This is presumably the cause of the changes in the rate of sodium excretion which occur with changes of posture (especially in an animal such as man who walks and stands in an upright posture). Standing up, which reduces the venous distention at the heart and in the head and neck and leads to a fall in arterial pressure, leads to a decreased rate of sodium ion excretion, and lying down to an increased excretion. Such alterations will produce short term fluctuations superimposed on the long term overall control of the extracellular fluid volume.

As mentioned above, this description of the mechanisms for regulating the volume of the extracellular fluid is probably far from complete. There is evidence that there are receptors which monitor the volume of the extracellular fluid independently of the plasma volume, and that there may be other hormonal systems besides aldosterone which regulate the rate of sodium excretion [16, 46].

4.4 *Limitations of the Equilibrium for Water and Salts*

The mechanisms outlined in the last two Sections maintain a very precise control over the volume and composition of the body fluids under a wide range of conditions of the environment and changes in the dietary intake of salts and water. The ability to maintain this constant internal environment in the face of changing circumstances depends very largely on the ability to alter the volume and solute content of the urine. Reduction of the available range of variations in the urine which can be produced, as may

occur in renal disease, reduces the range of circumstances over which the constancy of the internal environment may be maintained. The circumstances which may lead to appreciable changes in the internal environment, because the capacity of the regulatory mechanisms has been exceeded, can perhaps best be envisaged by considering the equilibrium which should normally exist for the input and output of salts and water. Consideration of this, together with the renal mechanisms for altering the volume and concentration of the urine, makes it possible to see the way in which the various mechanisms may interact with one another under circumstances which may overload one or more of the mechanisms. For a normal man, and for most other land mammals, overloading is most likely to occur when the amount of water (or rather less often salts) lost from the body exceeds the quantity available in the diet.

4.5 *Water Equilibrium*

The body's input of water is from two sources. One is the water present as water in the food and drink which is ingested, and the other is the water which is produced during the course of the metabolic breakdown of those substances which are used to provide the body's energy requirements. For most species, the first of these can in principle vary over a wide range, while the second is relatively constant and depends on the metabolic rate. Roughly 0.14 to 0.15 ml of water is produced for each kcal produced by metabolism, $(0.033 - 0.036 \text{ ml kJ}^{-1})$ the amount varying slightly with the substrate being used for metabolism. An active adult man whose metabolism is producing about 3000 kcal d^{-1} (12 600 kJ d^{-1}) will therefore synthesize $400 - 450$ ml of water, while at rest he will produce about 300 ml of water corresponding to about 2000 kcal d^{-1} (8400 kJ d^{-1}).

In addition to the more obviously fluid items of the diet, a good deal of water is contained in most commonly eaten foodstuffs, e.g. meat, potatoes etc. In this way an adult on a normal sort of Western mixed diet probably ingests about 750 ml of water,

apart from what is ingested in a fluid form.

Water is lost from the body by a number of routes. As well as the obvious form of fluid excreted as urine, water is also lost from the respiratory tract, the skin and the gastro-intestinal tract. Water is lost from the respiratory tract because man and many other animals exhale air which is near central body temperature and is saturated with water vapour. The air breathed in is usually cooler than body temperature and may or may not be saturated with water vapour, but will, under all tolerable environmental conditions, contain less water vapour than the expired air. This extra amount of water in the expired air is lost from the body, and the evaporation of this water (together with the warming of the inspired air) also involves the loss of some heat from the body. The actual quantity of water lost in this way will obviously depend on the temperature and humidity of the inspired air. The most that will be lost by an adult man at rest is about $350 - 400$ ml d^{-1}, this being the volume of water necessary to saturate at 37 °C a volume of dry air equal to the quantity exhaled during the day. If the air breathed in is at 20 °C (68 °F) and saturated with water vapour, the quantity of water lost will be reduced to $250 - 300$ ml.

The amount of water lost from the gastro-intestinal tract is usually quite small — the faeces contain somewhere around 150 ml d^{-1} for a normal man. It might be thought that this was water which had never been absorbed from the diet, but it is in fact the balance remaining after absorption of the water in the diet together with reabsorption of the water in the secretions of the gastro-intestinal tract. Under pathological conditions (e.g. diarrhoea or vomiting) some of these secretions are lost from the body, and under such circumstances the loss of water from the gastro-intestinal tract may be very much greater than the intake of water in the diet. (Since the digestive secretions also contain various ions, this will also have an effect on the salt balance and may affect the acid-base balance of the body — see below and Section 3.1).

The skin provides the route for a very variable and sometimes very large proportion of the total amount of water lost from the

body each day. Some water is always lost by this route in man, whatever the environmental circumstances, since some secretion of sweat and some diffusion of water through the skin always occurs. In addition to this 'basal' water loss, sweating is also a method of providing a moist skin surface from which water can evaporate. This allows heat to be disposed of as latent heat of evaporation (even when the air temperature is higher than the central body temperature). The amount of 'basal' water loss by a man is about 500 ml d^{-1}, and the amount of water lost to produce evaporative cooling depends on the amount of heat being generated (i.e. the metabolic rate) and the amount of heat that can be disposed of by radiation, conduction and convection, which in turn depends on the temperature of the environment. In a cold environment, it is not necessary to use evaporative cooling at all, unless vigorous exercise is being performed. However, when the environmental temperature is higher than body temperature, so that evaporative heat loss has to be used not only to remove all the metabolic heat, but also the heat gained from the environment by radiation, conduction or convection, more than 10 l of water per day may be lost in sweating. Although these figures apply to man, most mammals have somewhat similar problems, since even those which don't sweat use evaporation of water to keep themselves cool under hot conditions. A hot dog, for example, pants, which assists evaporation from the mucous membranes of its mouth and nose, while some other non-sweating animals spread saliva over their fur to provide a large area of damp surface from which water can evaporate.

A number of mammals which live in hot arid environments have special adaptations to enable them to reduce the amount of water which they need for cooling. Many small desert-dwelling animals largely avoid the problem by staying in deep burrows during the day and only coming out at night when the air temperature is lower than their body temperature. In the deep burrows, the temperature fluctuates little during the 24 hours and it is always cooler than the animal's body temperature. Some desert animals also reduce the water lost in the expired air by exhaling air which is saturated with water vapour, but cooled well below

body temperature [38]. This occurs because the blood supply to the nasal mucosa passes through an arrangement of small veins and arteries which acts as a heat exchanger. The venous blood which has been cooled as a result of the evaporation of water to saturate the inspired air cools the arterial blood which is on its way to the nasal mucosa. This means that the nasal mucosa remains cool until the air is breathed out again. The expired air is then recooled causing the water vapour to be recondensed where it is available for saturating the next breath. (This not only reduces the water lost in the expired air, but also the heat, so that more heat has to be disposed of by other routes). For almost all mammals, the total amount of air breathed has roughly the same relationship to the metabolic heat output (because the proportion of oxygen extracted is much the same). For an animal such as man, which breathes out air at, or only a little below, central body temperature, the amount of water lost in the expired air when breathing dry air is about the same as the amount of water produced by metabolism (see the figures above). The ability of some desert animals to breathe out air at a temperature considerably lower than their body temperature means that they lose less water in their expired air than they produce by metabolism (air saturated at 20 °C contains only about 1/3 the water vapour that air saturated at 37 °C contains), so that they are able to live entirely on dry food, and without drinking any water at all [37] (see also below).

Some large desert mammals, e.g. camels, avoid the necessity for using much water for evaporative cooling by not maintaining a constant body temperature [37]. During the day the body temperature rises when the environment is hotter than their body temperature, while during the night, when the environment is cooler than body temperature, they lose the heat gained during the day and cool down again. Some such animals, e.g. the oryx and some gazelles, can survive a rise of central body temperature (to over 46 °C [43]) which would be fatal for most mammals because of its effects on the brain. In these animals, although the central body temperature rises, the brain temperature does not, or at least rises much less. This is brought about by a

mechanism somewhat similar to that which enables small desert animals to breathe out air cooler than their central body temperature. In the oryx, the venous blood draining from the nasal mucosa, which has been cooled by the evaporation of water into the inspired air, enters a heat exchanger system (in this case an extension of the cavernous venous sinus) which, instead of cooling the arterial blood leading to the nasal mucosa, cools the blood in the numerous small arteries into which the internal carotid artery splits up in this species and which supply the blood to the brain [42]. This keeps the brain cooler than the central body temperature. (Although this mechanism is particularly well developed in desert dwelling animals such as the oryx, the majority of ungulates, e.g. sheep [3] also possess it).

4.6 *Regulation of Water Excretion by the Kidneys*

Water is lost by the routes described in the previous Section at a rate which depends largely upon environmental factors and which is not under direct physiological control. The rate at which water is excreted in the urine, however, can be very considerably altered by physiological mechanisms. The maximum amount depends on the volume of fluid entering the distal convoluted tubules, which in an adult man, amounts to about 15 ml min^{-1} or 20 l d^{-1} (and can under artificial conditions be even greater). For this reason it is extremely difficult to overload a normal healthy man with water, at least with fluids given by mouth, unless his physiological responses have been altered in some way, e.g. by injecting antidiuretic hormone. The minimum rate of water excretion depends on the quantity of solutes in the urine. With maximum secretion of antidiuretic hormone, the kidneys excrete as little water as their mode of operation permits. With a small solute load, the osmotic concentration of the urine is as high as the kidneys can make it. This, in man, is about 1400 mmol l^{-1}, but varies very much in different animals (with the lengths of their loops of Henle).

The process of making a concentrated urine involves the

reabsorption of water (without solutes) into the extracellular fluid of the renal medulla. The tubular fluid leaving the distal convoluted tubule is isotonic with the (cortical) plasma, so that the volume of water which is reabsorbed is the difference between the volume actually excreted and the volume that the solutes would have occupied at an osmotic pressure of $c.300$ mmol l^{-1}. The quantity of water reabsorbed must therefore increase as the quantity of solutes increases. This water tends to dilute the extra-cellular fluid of the renal medulla, and continuous activity by the loops of Henle is necessary to maintain the concentration gradient in the medulla. As the quantity of solutes increases the quantity of water entering the extracellular fluid of the medulla also increases and the maximum concentration difference which the loops of Henle are able to maintain falls. The osmotic con-centration of the extracellular fluid in the most central parts of the medulla must therefore fall and so the osmolar concentration of the urine also falls (see Fig. 11). This means that less water per unit of solute is reabsorbed, so that further increase in the quan-tity of solutes leads to a proportionally greater increase in the total volume of urine excreted. To illustrate this, suppose that the solute load is doubled. If the osmotic concentration of the urine remained the same, its volume would also double, but since the osmotic concentration falls, the volume increases by a factor of more than 2; in this example, if the osmotic concentration fell to 2/3 of its original value the volume would increase by a factor of 3.

There are a wide variety of substances which may be excreted in the urine, although only a few are normally present in the 'solute load' in sufficient quantity to be significant, at least as far as their effect on water balance is concerned. These substances include urea and various inorganic salts. Urea is derived from the deamination of amino acids, which occurs as a result of the break-down of protein. For a healthy person on a normal diet, the amount of urea produced depends on the amount of protein in the diet, but excretion of urea does not cease even if there is no protein in the diet (although it is considerably reduced — to about 5 g d^{-1} in man), since some amino acids are broken down in the

normal turnover of the body's structural proteins. (This state of affairs obviously cannot continue indefinitely, as the protein content of the body must be falling, so that the body is not in equilibrium, although it is possible to survive for several months on a protein-free diet). The quantities of inorganic salts in the urine depend very much on the quantities present in the diet and which have not left by other routes (see below).

For someone on a normal Western mixed diet the total quantity of solutes in the urine is unlikely to be less than about 700 mmol d^{-1}. This is made up of about 25 gm of urea which, since the molecular weight of urea is 60, represents 25/60 moles or 0.417 moles — say 0.400 moles. Since urea is not ionized this makes 400 mmol in solution. The remainder will be made up very largely of sodium, potassium, phosphate, sulphate and chloride ions, with relatively very small quantities of other ions and non-ionized substances. With this solute load, the maximum urinary osmotic concentration would be about 1200 mmol l^{-1}, so that the minimum volume of urine secreted per day will be about 580 ml.

On the basis of the above approximate figures, the minimum amount of water lost per day for a man at rest in a cool environment and on a normal diet will be about 500 ml through the skin, 350 ml through the respiratory system, 150 ml in the faeces and 600 ml in the urine, making a total of roughly 1600 ml. The amount gained will be about 350 ml from the synthesis of water during the breakdown of foodstuffs to provide energy and about 700 ml from the water in the diet. This leaves a deficit of about 550 ml which will usually be supplied in the form of drink. Note that (within the considerable margin of error in the figures quoted above) this is the minimum quantity of drink necessary to avoid a net loss of water during the day. Most people drink considerably more than this, in which case the output of urine will increase in parallel. On the other hand, increased water loss (usually as a result of an increased amount of heat to be got rid of by evaporation) will make it necessary to drink more than 550 ml of water so as to maintain water equilibrium. The increased breathing resulting from exercise has little effect on water balance in man, since the increased loss from the respiratory system is more or

less exactly balanced by the increased synthesis of water. Exercise does of course also increase the amount of heat to be disposed of and this usually does increase the net loss of water because of increased sweating.

If the intake of water is insufficient to balance the loss of water this leads to a reduction in the water content of the body fluids, but not (or at least a relatively smaller reduction) of the solute content. This means that the osmotic concentration of both the intracellular and extracellular fluid must rise, and its volume must fall. In the case of the extracellular fluid, this rise of osmotic concentration will be paralleled by a rise in the sodium (and chloride) concentration. Before any great change has occurred, thirst would be expected to cause an increase in the water intake to compensate for this, except in those incapable of voluntarily increasing their water intake (such as comatose patients or young babies).

For man under circumstances where fresh water is not readily available (e.g. when lost at sea after shipwrecks or in deserts) it can be seen from the preceding discussion that there are a number of possible ways of minimizing the water requirements. The most obvious way is by minimizing the amount of water needed for cooling, by reducing as far as possible the amount of heat needed to be disposed of by evaporation. This can be done by reducing the heat gained by radiation by keeping out of direct or reflected sunlight and by avoiding physical exertion when it is hot. In desert conditions, it is always much cooler at night — well below body temperature — so that if any exertion is necessary under such circumstances, this is the best time to undertake it. In warm weather at sea it is possible to cool oneself by pouring sea water on to the skin to provide water for evaporation or even to immerse oneself in the sea, which is always below central body temperature. The amount of water lost in the urine can be reduced to some extent by reducing the solute load. This can be done by eating a diet containing a minimal amount of, or even no, protein and a minimal amount of inorganic salts — certainly no more than is necessary to replace salts lost in the sweat. For some desert-living animals this is very important. For example, the kangaroo

rat can normally live without any water at all in its diet (except the small amount in dry seeds), but if fed on a diet containing large amounts of protein (more than about 40% of its energy supply) it can no longer do so, because the urine volume is increased due to the increased amount of urea excreted, and the water lost by evaporation and in the urine then exceeds the water gained from metabolism [37]. For man, whose urinary water loss is usually a much smaller proportion of the total water budget, this is somewhat less important (but can still make the difference between life and death for people who have been shipwrecked). However, it is still very important to minimize the solute load, and this is the reason why one should never drink sea-water when fresh water is in short supply. The osmotic concentration of sea-water is about 1200 mmol l^{-1} (mostly in the form of sodium chloride) which is slightly less than the maximum concentration which healthy human kidneys can produce. However, if say, 500 ml (approx. 1 pint) of sea-water is drunk in a day, this contains 600 mmol of solutes which must be excreted again via the kidneys. This together with the normal daily load of solutes (say another 600 mmol) makes a total of 1200 mmol d^{-1}. The highest concentration that the kidneys can produce when the urine contains such a large quantity of solutes is somewhere in the region of 1000 mmol l^{-1} (see Section 2.9), so that the total volume of urine will be 1.2 litres. This means that drinking 500 ml of sea-water has increased the urine volume by about 700 ml (from approximately 500 to 1200 ml) producing a net loss of 200 ml of water. Drinking larger volumes of sea-water will increase the solute load even more and further reduce the final concentration of the urine, so producing proportionally larger net losses of water. (Apart from this, drinking sea-water produces a rapid rise in the osmotic concentration of the extracellular fluid, as the very hypertonic fluid in the stomach and small intestine draws water osmotically out of the cells and thence from the extracellular fluid. This in turn increases the osmotic concentration of the extracellular fluid, thus further aggravating the effects of the reduction of water content of the body and exacerbating the sensation of thirst. The magnesium and sulphate ions in sea-water

are also likely to produce diarrhoea. Although this applies to man, animals such as the kangaroo rat, whose maximum urinary concentration is about 6000 mmol l^{-1}, can drink sea-water with impunity and thereby obtain a net gain of water.)

4.7 Equilibrium for Salts

All the salts which enter the body are taken in by mouth (unless experimentally or therapeutically injected). Although a large range of salts and inorganic ions are present in the diet, and the regulation of the body's content of the various ions involved may be very important, the discussion will be mainly restricted to those which are present in large quantities in the body or the urine, or which have special significance to the problems of maintaining the constancy of the internal environment. Inorganic ions which are present in large quantities in the body include sodium, potassium, chloride, bicarbonate and phosphate ions. Ions of special significance for the maintenance of the internal environment include hydrogen ions, which have already been dealt with, and sometimes sulphate ions. There are many other ions which are of great importance in the body (e.g. magnesium and calcium ions). However, the amount of any of these ions which appears in the urine is usually relatively small and therefore has little effect either on the total solute content or on the anion-cation balance of the urine.

Of the ions mentioned above (i.e. Na^+, K^+, Cl^-, HCO_3^-, HPO_4^{--} and SO_4^{--}), sodium, potassium and chloride ions will for the moment be considered together. These are all present in the body in large quantities, nearly all in solution in the body fluids. These ions are absorbed almost entirely as the ions themselves rather than in combination and make up the majority of the inorganic ions in the 'salts' in a normal diet.

A significant part of the total number of solute particles, particularly in the extracellular fluid, is made up of bicarbonate ions. Changes in the bicarbonate concentrations of body fluids are associated with changes in the acid-base equilibrium of the

body, and have been dealt with already. However, bicarbonate ions are also involved in the salt and water equilibrium of the body and so will also be mentioned below where appropriate.

Although phosphate and sulphate normally form quite a substantial part of the total number of anions in the urine, they are mostly derived from metabolic breakdown of substances which are present in the diet and only to a small extent absorbed as the ions themselves. (Indeed, sulphate ions even if present in the diet are very poorly absorbed, hence the effectiveness of the old fashioned 'purges', sodium sulphate or magnesium sulphate.) Although the rate of excretion of these two ions depends on the amount of their precursors absorbed from the diet, this does not depend on the 'salt' content of the diet. All that is absorbed, however, has to leave again via the kidneys since they provide the only route by which any significant quantity of either of these ions leave the body.

These inorganic ions all leave the body in the urine, and sodium, potassium, chloride and bicarbonate ions also leave in varying amounts via the gastro-intestinal tract and the skin. In the case of these four ions, any which are lost via the gastro-intestinal tract are ions that have not been reabsorbed from intestinal secretions rather than ions which have not been absorbed in the first place. The quantity of ions lost by this route is normally quite small, but (as for water) may be greatly increased in some illnesses. The secretions in different parts of the gastro-intestinal tract differ markedly in their composition. They all have an osmotic concentration fairly similar to that of the extra-cellular fluid, but (partly as a result of their mucus content) a relatively higher potassium concentration and lower sodium concentration. The gastric secretions are highly acid — so acid, in fact, that hydrogen ions make up a majority of the cations, the only body fluid for which this is true — while the secretions in the small intestine (pancreatic juice, bile, succus entericus, etc.) are alkaline. This means that loss of gastric secretions, e.g. by vomiting, causes a loss of water and salts and also tends to make the extra-cellular fluid more alkaline, since the fluid lost from the body is acid. If, on the other hand, duodenal secretions are lost in large

quantities, as in severe diarrhoea or with aspiration of duodenal contents, water and salts are again lost but the extracellular fluid tends to become more acid. Under normal circumstances, the loss of ions from the gastro-intestinal tract is small, amounting to less than 5 mmol d^{-1} of each of the ions under consideration (for man).

The picture is somewhat different when the loss from the skin is considered. The sweat consists essentially of a solution of sodium chloride (with some potassium chloride) which is considerably hypotonic to the extracellular fluid. The actual concentration of sodium chloride varies considerably from one person to another and from time to time but is usually around 1/4 − 1/3 of that in the extracellular fluid, making in rough round figures a concentration of about 40 mmol l^{-1} for both sodium and chloride ions. The potassium concentration is also very variable, but is usually about 1/10 of the sodium concentration [19]. This means that the minimum loss of sodium and chloride ions in the sweat is at least 20 mmol d^{-1} (500 ml of water containing 40 mmol l^{-1} of each). The maximum loss is more than 400 mmol d^{-1} of each (contained in 10 l of sweat), representing more than 10% of the total body content of sodium chloride. The potassium loss in the sweat is much less than for either of the above ions, and will range between about 2 and 50 mmol d^{-1}. Phosphate and sulphate ions (once they or their precursors have been absorbed) are not secreted in significant quantities either into the gastro-intestinal secretions or in the sweat, and the same quantity as that which is absorbed must appear in the urine, if the quantity in the body is to remain constant. The mechanisms which regulate the body's content of these two ions operate independently of each other and of the regulation of the other ions which are under consideration.

4.8 Excretion of Inorganic Ions in the Urine

The urine contains a number of different ions, and as in any other solution, the total number of anions must be the same as the total number of cations. The anions which may be present in

quantity include phosphate, sulphate, chloride and bicarbonate ions, while the cations are sodium and potassium ions, together with ammonium ions. Taking the anions first, the rate of excretion of phosphate and sulphate ions depends on the quantities of these ions and of their precursors which have been absorbed from the gastro-intestinal tract. The concentration of bicarbonate varies inversely with the hydrogen ion concentration, so that the quantity of bicarbonate excreted depends on both the volume and the hydrogen ion concentration of the urine. These anions must be balanced by an equivalent number of cations.

For the cations, (sodium and potassium ions will, for the moment, be considered together) the quantities of sodium and potassium ions which should be excreted depend on the balance remaining from those absorbed, after the losses in the sweat and from the gastro-intestinal tract have been taken into account. If this quantity is less than the quantity of anions (i.e. sulphate, phosphate and bicarbonate) in the urine (after allowing for hydrogen and ammonium ions — see below) then more cations are needed to balance the remaining anions, and more sodium and/or potassium ions will be lost from the body than have been absorbed. If, on the other hand, this quantity is greater than the quantity of anions, then chloride ions (in company with which sodium ions are absorbed from a normal sort of diet) will be excreted. This means that there is a lower limit for the loss of cations in the urine which is set by the quantity of anions. This occurs because the distal tubules and collecting ducts are not permeable to sulphate and phosphate ions, nor are they able to actively reabsorb these ions, so that the quantity appearing in the urine is the same as the quantity entering the distal convoluted tubules. The presence of these ions in the tubules prevents further active net reabsorption of cations once all the diffusible anions (i.e. chloride ions) have been (passively) reabsorbed. Transport of further cations will generate an increased electrical potential (with the inside of the tubule negative) which makes them diffuse back as fast as they can be transported. Under these circumstances the urine will effectively be free of all diffusible anions since the potential gradient generated will drive them out of the tubule.

The absence of chloride ions in the urine is therefore a good indicator that the kidneys are transporting sodium and potassium ions out of the tubules as hard as they can, which normally indicates that the body is suffering (or has suffered) a net loss of sodium and/or potassium ions.

The actual minimum quantities of cations which must be excreted will depend not only on the quantities of phosphate and sulphate ions excreted but also on the pH or, rather on what might be called the hydrogen ion content of the urine. (The hydrogen ion content of the urine is the number of hydrogen ions which are being excreted, i.e. the titratable acid, plus the ammonia content.) When the hydrogen ion content of the urine is high, the number of anions which must be neutralized by cations is reduced because of 3 different factors. Some of the hydrogen ions form carbon dioxide and water by combining with bicarbonate ions; they are therefore no longer present as anions. Other hydrogen ions combine with divalent phosphate ions to form monovalent phosphate ions, in the course of the phosphate ions' buffering action:

$$HPO_4^{--} + H^+ \rightleftharpoons H_2PO_4^- \qquad (4.1)$$

which further reduces the anionic charges which have to be neutralized. Thus, for both phosphate and bicarbonate ions the number of anionic charges to be neutralized depends on the final pH of the urine. The third factor depends on the ammonium concentration of the urine. As mentioned above (Section 2.10), circumstances which lead to the excretion of an acid urine also lead to increased synthesis of ammonia by the cells of the distal convoluted tubules and collecting ducts and hence to an increased excretion of ammonium ions in the urine. Each ammonium ion is a cation and can therefore balance an anion. It also represents a hydrogen ion which has combined with an ammonia molecule, so that it contributes to the final hydrogen ion content of the urine, but not to its hydrogen ion concentration. The actual hydrogen ion concentration of the urine is so low that hydrogen ions as such make a negligible contribution. A day's output of urine (say 2 litres), even with a pH of 4.4 ($[H^+] = 4 \times 10^{-5}$) contains only 8×10^{-5} Eq or 0.08 mEq of free hydrogen ions.

For a normal man on a mixed diet, phosphorus and sulphur are absorbed in sufficient quantities to require the excretion of about 50 mmol of phosphate and 25 mmol of sulphate ions per day. The pK representing the equilibrium constant for the reaction of phosphate ions represented by equation (4.1) is about 6.8, so that at a pH of 7.4 approximately 4/5 of the phosphate ions are in the divalent form (HPO_4^{--}) and 1/5 in the monovalent form ($H_2PO_4^-$). The 50 mmol will therefore have about 90 mEq of anionic charges. The sulphate ions are all divalent, so have 50 mEq of anionic charges. If the urinary pH is 7.4, its bicarbonate concentration will be about 24 mEq l^{-1}, so, assuming a urine output of 1.5 litres d^{-1}, the total quantity of bicarbonate will be 36 mEq (1.5 × 24). Thus the total anionic charges are:

Phosphate	90
Sulphate	50
Bicarbonate	36
	$\overline{176}$ mEq d^{-1}

This must be balanced by (very nearly) the same number of cationic charges on sodium and potassium ions (since the production of ammonia with such a urine pH will normally be very small). If, on the other hand, the urine has a pH of 4.4, more than 99% of the phosphate ions will be in the monovalent ($H_2PO_4^-$) form, so will represent only 50 mEq, the sulphate ions will still represent (very nearly) 50 mEq and the bicarbonate concentration will be only about 0.024 mEq l^{-1}, so that the anionic charges will be:

Phosphate	50
Sulphate	50
Bicarbonate	0
	$\overline{100}$ mEq d^{-1}

The ammonia production under these circumstances may be such that well over 100 mEq d^{-1} of ammonium ions are excreted in the urine, which means that there is no necessity to excrete any sodium or potassium ions at all in order to balance the anions which are excreted. Thus, the hydrogen ion content of the urine and hence the state of the acid-base equilibrium of the body may

have a considerable effect on the number of sodium and potassium ions which are necessarily excreted in the urine. Indeed, when the body is depleted of potassium ions, an inappropriately acid urine is often secreted (see Section 3.6), because the pH inside the cells of the tubules is lower than normal. This has the effect of reducing the rate of loss of potassium ions in the urine, since the tubule cells secrete hydrogen ions into the urine, so increasing its hydrogen ion content and thus reducing the number of other cations which must be excreted.

4.9 Regulation of Renal Excretion of Sodium and Potassium Ions

In the previous chapter, sodium and potassium ions were considered together, but the quantity of each excreted in the urine can be altered independently within the limitations set by the sum of their quantities being not less than the number necessary to balance the charges on the non-reabsorbable anions being excreted.

In the proximal convoluted tubules, nearly all the potassium ions which have entered the glomerular filtrate are reabsorbed. In the distal convoluted tubules, more sodium ions are reabsorbed and some potassium ions re-enter the tubular fluid [4]. The rate at which sodium ions are transported out of the distal tubules depends on the rate at which they diffuse into the tubular cells. This diffusion increases with increase in the concentration of aldosterone circulating in the blood, since this affects the cells in such a way that the permeability to sodium ions of the tubular walls of the cells is increased. As in any other cell, diffusion of sodium ions into the cell will usually be associated with passive diffusion of potassium ions out (even if not in a 1 to 1 ratio). The sodium ions are actively extruded both into the tubules and into the extracellular fluid (again in exchange for potassium ions) with the result that there is a net transfer of sodium ions from the tubule to the extracellular fluid. (See Section 2.8). In the proximal tubules, the potassium ions which diffuse out of the cells into the tubules, together with those originally in the glomerular filtrate,

are re-absorbed by the tubular cells (and passively diffuse out
into the extracellular fluid). To maintain electrical balance, this
transfer of cations out of the tubules must be associated with
the transfer of an equivalent number of anions — in this case,
mostly chloride ions, which passively diffuse down their electrochemical gradient, and bicarbonate ions, which are transported
indirectly as a result of hydrogen in secretion. In the distal tubule,
similar ionic movements occur, but when there are no more
anions (which can be re-absorbed), present in the tubules, it is
no longer possible to transport potassium ions from the tubules
into the cells. However, if the tubular walls of the tubular cells
are relatively permeable to sodium ions, sodium ions will still
diffuse into the cells down their electrochemical gradient, in
which case potassium ions must diffuse out and there must, in
this case, be in effect a 1 to 1 exchange of sodium and potassium
ions even though active reabsorption of potassium ions is still
taking place [31]. This means that under circumstances when
the kidneys are extracting as many sodium and potassium ions
as possible from the urine, an increased secretion of aldosterone
will still reduce the number of sodium ions lost in the urine but
at the expense of an equivalent increase in the loss of potassium
ions. Indeed, the action of aldosterone in sufficient quantities
can lead to a reduction in the rate of loss of sodium ions in the
urine to a very low level (somewhere around 1 mEq l^{-1} [30]), at
the expense of an increase in the loss of potassium ions. This
happens even when the body is deficient in potassium ions as
well as sodium ions.

The quantity of fluid entering the distal tubules of an adult
man is about 20 l d^{-1} and this has a sodium concentration of
about 75 mEq l^{-1}, making approximately 1500 mEq d^{-1} of
sodium ions. In the absence of aldosterone, the permeability to
sodium ions of the walls of the distal convoluted tubules is
relatively low, but even so, a considerable reabsorption of sodium
ions from the tubular fluid always occurs — in man at least half
of the sodium ions entering the distal tubules are reabsorbed.
This means that the maximum rate of sodium excretion for a man
is very roughly 750 mEq d^{-1}. In animals with a very labile

glomerular filtration rate, such as the dog, the quantity of sodium ions entering the distal tubules may increase greatly when the glomerular filtration rate is increased, and although the actual number of sodium ions reabsorbed may not change, it will be a smaller proportion of the quantity arriving at the distal tubules. Such animals can tolerate a proportionally much higher sodium chloride intake than man, provided they have access to sufficient water to replace the volume of urine necessary to dissolve the sodium chloride as it is re-excreted.

For man, the absolute minimum rate at which sodium ions leave the body is about 30 mEq d^{-1} made up of 5 mEq in the faeces, about $1 - 2$ mEq in the urine and about 20 mEq in the sweat. This is considerably less than the quantity present in a normal Western diet, and any sodium ions in excess of this minimum will be excreted in the urine. The rate of sodium loss in a healthy individual is increased by an increase in the rate of sweating and may rise to over 400 mEq d^{-1} with physical exertion in a hot environment (see above) and this is more than the sodium content of a normal diet. This (net) sodium chloride loss is of course associated with loss of water, and since the sweat is hypotonic to the extracellular fluid, tends to raise the osmotic concentration of the extracellular fluid. However, if sufficient water is drunk to replace the volume of sweat lost, the effect is (nearly) equivalent to a loss of sodium chloride alone. Under such circumstances, the osmotic concentration of the extracellular fluid will be maintained (by adjustment of the rate of secretion of antidiuretic hormone), so that the volume of the extracellular fluid will fall. This will stimulate the secretion of aldosterone so that the kidneys do their best to prevent the loss of sodium ions in the urine, but this cannot restore the sodium ion content of the body unless the intake can be made to exceed the rate of loss. The lowered volume of the extracellular fluid creates a sensation of thirst in man but, rather curiously, not always an increased appetite for salt. Many animals have much better mechanisms than man for regulating their sodium salt intake to their requirements [15]. People who start to live and work in very hot environments have to remember to increase their salt intake, at least for

a considerable period of time until they get into the habit of eating more salt, otherwise they will suffer 'heat exhaustion' and muscle cramps etc [28]. This has been found to be particularly important for athletes taking part in competitions in hotter climates than they are accustomed to, partly because they often have little time to become accustomed to the hotter environment [11]. The effects of salt depletion leading to an increased and apparently insatiable thirst have been very well described by Heyerdahl in his account of the Kon-Tiki Expedition [23].

The minimum loss of potassium ions is comparable with that of sodium ions − roughly 30 mEq d^{-1}, consisting of about 5 mEq in the faeces, less than 5 mEq in the sweat and about 20 mEq in the urine. However, unlike sodium ions, the minimum rate of potassium ion excretion in the urine varies very much more with the other constituents of the urine. An alkaline urine and a low rate of sodium ion excretion (or rather, a high level of circulating aldosterone) both lead to an increased rate of potassium excretion, as described above. Even so, the normal dietary intake of potassium is well above the minimum loss and, as with sodium ions, any excess is excreted in the urine. The rate of potassium loss is increased very much less by increased sweating than is the sodium loss, so that a healthy individual should not become potassium deficient in the normal course of events. However, a good deal of potassium may be lost from the body in illness − e.g., prolonged or severe diarrhoea or diabetes (Section 3.5) − following which it may take a long time to replace the potassium on the normal dietary intake. During this period, hydrogen ions are excreted in the urine in inappropriate quantities, because of the low intra-cellular pH in the tubular cells (Section 3.6) and this reduces the potassium excretion. Provided the rate of loss is now less than the rate at which potassium ions are being absorbed from the diet, the deficiency of potassium will eventually be made up.

Appendix
Membrane Potentials

1. *Membrane Potentials*

For any voltage (V) and resistance (R) the current (I) that flows can be calculated from the relationship known as Ohms law.

$$I = \frac{V}{R}$$

Here, it is more convenient to use the conductivity (C) (which is the reciprocal of the resistance), instead of the resistance. In this case:

$$I = VC$$

For any ion passing through a membrane, the conductivity, which is a measure of the current which flows for a unit applied voltage, will depend both on the permeability of the membrane to that particular ion and on the concentration of the ion. (Obviously no current will pass if the membrane is not permeable to a particular ion, and also no current will flow, however permeable the membrane is, if there are no ions to pass through.) In the cell membrane, the permeabilities to the flow of sodium and potassium ions are very different while their concentrations are fairly similar. Hence the conductivities for the two ions must be different.

For potassium ions, the voltage driving the 'potassium current' is the difference between the equilibrium potential for potassium ions and the actual membrane potential. Thus:

$$I_K = (E_K - E_m)C_K \tag{1}$$

(where E_m is the membrane potential, and the subscripts represent the values of current, etc. relating to the flow of potassium ions).

Similarly for sodium ions,

$$I_{Na} = (E_{Na} - E_m)C_{Na} \qquad (2)$$

When the sodium pump is not active the membrane potential changes only very slowly so there can be no net movement of charge through the membrane. The currents carried by the sodium and the potassium ions must be equal and opposite, so that:

$$I_K = -I_{Na}$$

Substituting the values from equations (1) and (2),

$$(E_K - E_m)C_K = -(E_{Na} - E_m)C_{Na}$$

Multiplying out the brackets,

$$E_K C_K - E_m C_K = -E_{Na} C_{Na} + E_m C_{Na}$$

Collecting together the terms with E_m in them onto the left hand side,

$$E_m C_K + E_m C_{Na} = E_K C_K + E_{Na} C_{Na}$$

Extracting E_m,

$$E_m(C_K + C_{Na}) = E_K C_K + E_{Na} C_{Na}$$

so that,

$$E_m = \frac{E_K C_K + E_{Na} C_{Na}}{C_K + C_{Na}} \qquad (3)$$

which enables the actual value of the membrane potential to be calculated, provided enough of the quantities on the right hand side are known. In fact, it is only necessary to know the equilibrium potentials (or concentration ratios, from which the equilibrium potentials can be calculated by using the Nernst equation – see Section 1.8) for sodium and potassium ions, and the ratio of their conductivities. (The ratio is all that is needed as the conductivities appear in both top and bottom of the right hand side, so that multiplying them both by any constant will have no effect on the membrane potential since the constant will always cancel out.) From the form of the right hand side of the equation, it can be seen that the membrane potential must always lie somewhere between the sodium and the potassium equilibrium

potentials and that it will lie nearest to the equilibrium potential of the ion with the greater conductivity. If the conductivities are equal, the equation reduces to $E_m = (E_K + E_{Na})/2$, i.e. the membrane potential is halfway between the two equilibrium potentials, while if the potassium conductivity is 100 times the sodium conductivity, then $E_m = (100E_K + E_{Na})/101$, and the sodium equilibrium potential has very little effect on the membrane potential.

2. Calculation of Passive Membrane Potentials

The equilibrium potential for any ion can be calculated from the Nernst equation. E.g. for potassium

$$E_K = \frac{RT}{F} \log_e \frac{[K_o^+]}{[K_i^+]}$$

(where the subscript o and i represent the concentration outside and inside the cell respectively). The logarithm to base e of a number is always 2.3026 times bigger than its logarithm to base 10 (since $\log_e (10)$ is 2.3026). By combining this constant with R, T and F, the Nernst equation for potassium ions (or any other univalent ion) can be written as

$$E_K = 58.0 \cdot \log_{10} \frac{[K_o^+]}{[K_i^+]} \text{ mV (at 25 °C)}$$

This means that a 10 : 1 concentration ratio for any ion corresponds to a membrane potential of 58 mV. (This is therefore the voltage change that a pH meter should register corresponding to a change in pH of 1 unit — see Section 1.4).

Taking the intracellular : extracellular concentration ratio for potassium ions to be 15 : 1, then

$$E_K = 58.0 \cdot \log_{10} (1/15) \text{ mV} = -67.2 \text{ mV}$$

If the concentration ratio for sodium ions is 1 : 10, then the equilibrium potential for sodium ions is + 58.0 mV. Assuming a conductance ratio of 50 : 1 in favour of potassium ions, the membrane

potential will be

$$E_m = \frac{-67.2 \times 50 + 58.0 \times 1}{51} \text{ mV}$$

$$= -64.7 \text{ mV}$$

which is only 2.5 mV from the potassium equilibrium potential, but 122.7 mV from the sodium equilibrium potential.

If the conductance ratio were only 10 : 1 then,

$$E_m = \frac{-67.2 \times 10 + 58.0 \times 1}{11} \text{ mV}$$

$$= -55.8 \text{ mV}$$

or 11.4 mV from the potassium equilibrium potential.

3. Membrane Potentials with the Sodium Pump Active

With the sodium pump active, the cell is in equilibrium and the membrane potential stays constant, so no net movement either of charge or of individual ion species can be taking place. The pump transports more sodium ions out than potassium ions in, in a ratio that we will assume is 3 : 2. This means that the passive diffusion of sodium ions in and potassium ions out must also be in the ratio of 3 : 2. Equation (3) is no longer applicable, since the rates of diffusion are no longer equal. However, the currents due to the different ions are still given by equations (1) and (2). Now

$$3I_K = 2(-I_{Na})$$

so that substituting the values from equations (1) and (2)

$$3(E_K - E_m)C_K = -2(E_{Na} - E_m)C_{Na}$$

Solving this for E_m in the same way as that used to produce equation (3)

$$E_m = \frac{3(E_K)C_K + 2(E_{Na})C_{Na}}{3C_K + 2C_{Na}}$$

Substituting the values of the equilibrium potentials used above

and using a 50 : 1 ratio of the conductivities,

$$E_m = \frac{3(-67.2)50 + 2(58.0)1}{3.50 + 2.1} \, mV$$

$$= -65.6 \, mV$$

In this case the activity of the sodium pump has increased the membrane potential by 0.9 mV.

4. Effect of Sodium Pump with a low Potassium : Sodium Permeability Ratio

If the permeability ratio is only 10 : 1 then

$$E_m = \frac{(3(-67.2)10) + (2(58.0)1)}{3.10 + 2.1} \, mV$$

$$= -59.4 \, mV$$

so that (comparing this with the value found above) the activity of the pump has increased the membrane potential by 3.6 mV.

Suggestions
for Further Reading

Black, D.A.K. (1968) *Essentials of Fluid Balance* (Ed. 4)
Blackwell Scientific Publications, Oxford (Deals with disturbances of the internal environment from a clinical point of view)

Pitts, R.F. (1968) *Physiology of the Kidneys and Body Fluids* (Ed. 2)
Year Book Medical Publishers, Chicago (A detailed review of the whole of renal physiology)

Robinson, J.R. (1972) *Fundamentals of Acid-Base Regulation* (Ed. 4)
Blackwell Scientific Publications, Oxford (Covers in considerable detail the basic chemistry and physiology of disturbances of acid-base equilibrium)

References

1. Addis, T. and Drury, D.R. (1923), The Rate of Urea Excretion, V. The Effect of Changes in Blood Urea Concentration on the Rate of Urea Excretion, *J. Biol. Chem.*, 55, 105–111.
2. Van Assendelft, O.W., Mook, G.A. and Zylstra, W.G. (1973), International System of Units (SI) in Physiology, *Pflugers Arch.* 339, 265–272.
3. Baker, M.A. and Hayward, J.N. (1968), The Influence of the Nasal Mucosa and the Carotid Rete upon Hypothalamic Temperature in Sheep, *J. Physiol. (Lond.)* 198, 561–579.
4. Berliner, R.W. (1960), Renal Mechanism for Potassium Excretion, *Harvey Lect.* 55, 141–171.
5. Berliner, R.W., Levinsky, N.G., Davidson, D.G. and Eden, M. (1958), Dilution and Concentration of the Urine and the Action of Antidiuretic Hormone, *Amer. J. Med.* 24, 730–744.
6. Bernard, C. (1885), *Leçons sur les phénomenes de la vie communs aux animaux et aux végétaux.* Ballière, Paris.
7. Bloom, W.D. and Fawcett, D.W. (1968), *A Textbook of Histology* (9th Ed.). W.B. Saunders, Philadelphia.
8. Boulpaep, E.L. and Seely, J.F. (1971), Electrophysiology of Proximal and Distal Tubules in the Autoperfused Dog Kidney, *Amer. J. Physiol.* 221, 1084–1096.
9. Burg, M.B. and Grantham, J.J. (1971), In: *Membranes and Ion Transport. Vol. 3.* Ed: E.E. Bittar. Wiley-Interscience, London, pp 49–78.
10. Campbell, E.J.M. (1962), RIpH, *Lancet*, 1, 681–683.
11. Clarkson, E.M., Curtis, J.R., Jewkes, R.J., Jones, B.E., Luck, V.A., De Wardener, H.E. and Phillips, N. (1971), Slow Sodium. An Oral Slowly Released Sodium Chloride Preparation, *Brit. Med. J.* 3, 604–607.
12. Coulson, R.A., Hernandez, T. and Dessauer, H.G. (1950), Alkaline Tide of the Alligator. *Proc. Soc. Exp. Biol. Med.* 74, 866–869.

159

160 THE KIDNEYS AND THE INTERNAL ENVIRONMENT

13. Coxon, R.V. and Kay, R.H. (1967), *A Primer of General Physiology*. Butterworths, London.

14. Creese, R., Neil, M.W., Ledingham, J.M. and Vere, D.W. (1962), The Terminology of Acid-Base Regulation, *Lancet* 1, 419—421.

15. Denton, D.A. (1965), Evolutionary Aspects of the Emergence of Aldosterone Secretion and Salt Appetite, *Physiol. Rev.* 45, 245—295.

16. Dirks, J.H., Cirksena, W.J. and Berliner, R.W. (1965), The Effect of Saline Infusion on Sodium Reabsorption by the Proximal Tubule in the Dog, *J. Clin. Invest.* 44, 1160—1170.

17. Dyball, R.E.J. (1971), Oxytocin and ADH Secretion in Relation to Electrical Activity in Antidromically Identified Supraoptic and Paraventricular Neurones, *J. Physiol. (Lond.)* 214, 245—256.

18. Fitzsimons, J.T. (1972), Thirst, *Physiol. Rev.* 52, 468—561.

19. Furman, K.I. and Beer, G. (1963), Dynamic Changes in Sweat Electrolyte Composition induced by Heat Stress as an Indication of Acclimatization and Aldosterone Activity, *Clin. Sci.* 24, 7—12.

20. Geibisch, G., Berger, L. and Pitts, R.F. (1955), The Extrarenal Response to Acute Acid-Base Disturbances of Respiratory Origin, *J. Clin. Invest.* 34, 231—245.

21. Geibisch, G., Malnic, G., Klose, R.M. and Windhager, E.E. (1966), Effect of Ionic Substitutions on Distal Potential Differences in Rat Kidney, *Amer. J. Physiol.* 211, 560—568.

22. Hervey, G.R., McCance, R.A. and Tayler, R.G.O. (1946), Forced Diuresis during Hydropenia, *Nature* 157, 338.

23. Heyerdahl, T. (1950), *The Kon-Tiki Expedition*. George Allen and Unwin, London. (Chapter V).

24. Horster, M. and Thurau, K. (1968), Micropuncture Studies on the Filtration Rate of Single Superficial and Juxtamedullary Glomeruli in the Rat Kidney, *Pflügers Arch.* 301, 162—181.

25. Hunt, J.N. (1956), The Influence of Dietary Sulphur on the Urinary Output of Acid in Man. *Clin. Sci.* 15, 119—134.

26. Keynes, R.D. (1954), The Ionic Fluxes in Frog Muscle, *Proc. Roy. Soc. B.* 142, 359—382.

27. Keynes, R.D. and Maisel, G.W. (1954), The Energy Requirement for Sodium Extrusion from a Frog Muscle, *Proc. Roy. Soc. B.* 142, 383—392.

28. King, B.A. and Barry, M.E. (1962), The Physiological Adaptations to Heat-Stress with a Classification of Heat Illness and a Description of the Features of Heat Exhaustion, *South African Med. J.* 36, 451—455.

29. Landes, R.R., Leonhardt, K.O. and Duruman, N. (1964), A Clinical Study of the Oxygen Tension of the Urine and Renal Structures. II. *J. Urol.* **92**, 171–178.
30. Malnic, G., Klose, R.M. and Geibisch, G. (1966), Micropuncture Study of Distal Tubular Potassium and Sodium in the Rat Nephron. *Amer. J. Physiol.* **211**, 529–547.
31. Malnic, G., Klose, R.M. and Geibisch, G. (1966), Microperfusion Studies of Distal Tubular Potassium and Sodium Transfer in Rat Kidney, *Amer. J. Physiol.* **211**, 548–559.
32. Müller, E., McIntosh, J.F. and van Slyke, D.D. (1928), Studies of urea excretion. II. Relationship between Urine Volume and the Rate of Urea Excretion by Normal Adults, *J. Clin. Invest.* **6**, 427–465.
33. Pappenheimer, J.R. and Kinter, W.B. (1956), Haematocrit Ratio of Blood within Mammalian Kidney and its Significance for Renal Haemodynamics, *Amer. J. Physiol.* **185**, 377–390.
34. Rapoport, S., Brodsky, W.A., West, C.D. and Mackler, B. (1949), Urinary Flow and Excretion of Solutes During Osmotic Diuresis in Hydropenic Man, *Amer. J. Physiol.* **156**, 433–442.
35. Ross, E.J. and Christie, S.B.M. (1969), Hypernatremia, *Medicine* **48**, 441–473.
36. Schmidt-Nielsen, B. and O'Dell, R. (1961), Structure and Concentrating Mechanism in the Mammalian Kidney, *Amer. J. Physiol.* **200**, 1119–1124.
37. Schmidt-Nielsen, K. (1964). *Desert Animals. Physiological Problems of Heat and Water.* Oxford University Press, Oxford.
38. Schmidt-Nielsen, K. (1972). *How Animals Work.* Cambridge University Press, Cambridge.
39. Schmidt-Nielsen, K., Schmidt-Nielsen, B., Jarnum, S.A. and Houpt, T.R. (1957). Body Temperature of the Camel and its Relation to Water Economy, *Amer. J. Physiol.* **188**, 103–112.
40. Schnermann, J., Wright, F.S., Davis, J.M., von Stackelberg, W. and Grill, G. (1970), Regulation of Superficial Nephron Filtration Rate by Tubulo-Glomerular Feedback, *Pflügers Arch.* **318**, 147–175.
41. Smith, H.W. (1951). *The Kidney: Structure and Function in Health and Disease.* Oxford University Press, New York.
42. Taylor, C.R. (1969), The Eland and the Oryx. *Scientific American.* **220** (January), 88–97.
43. Taylor, C.R. (1970), Dehydration and Heat: Effects on Temperature Regulation of East African Ungulates, *Amer. J. Physiol.* **219**, 1136–1139.

44. Thomas, R.C. (1972), Electrogenic Sodium Pump in Nerve and Muscle Cells, *Physiol. Rev.* **52**, 563—594.
45. Waddel, W.J. and Bates, R.G. (1969), Intracellular pH, *Physiol. Rev.* **49**, 285—329.
46. De Wardener, H.E. (1969), Control of Sodium Reabsorption, *Brit. Med. J.* **3**, 611—616 and 676—683.
47. Wilde, W.S. and Varburger, C. (1967), Albumen Multiplier in Kidney Vasa Recta analysed by Microspectrophotometry of T-1824, *Amer. J. Physiol.* **213**, 1233—1243.

Index

Index

165